Delivering Person-Centred Care in Nursing

Sara Miller McCune founded SAGE Publishing in 1965 to support the dissemination of usable knowledge and educate a global community. SAGE publishes more than 1000 journals and over 800 new books each year, spanning a wide range of subject areas. Our growing selection of library products includes archives, data, case studies and video. SAGE remains majority owned by our founder and after her lifetime will become owned by a charitable trust that secures the company's continued independence.

Los Angeles | London | New Delhi | Singapore | Washington DC | Melbourne

Delivering Person-Centred Care in Nursing

2E

Bob Price

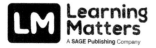

Learning Matters
A SAGE Publishing Company
1 Oliver's Yard
55 City Road
London EC1Y 1SP

SAGE Publications Inc.
2455 Teller Road
Thousand Oaks, California 91320

SAGE Publications India Pvt Ltd
B 1/I 1 Mohan Cooperative Industrial Area
Mathura Road
New Delhi 110 044

SAGE Publications Asia-Pacific Pte Ltd
3 Church Street
#10-04 Samsung Hub
Singapore 049483

© Bob Price 2022

First published 2019

Second edition 2022

Editor: Laura Walmsley
Development Editor: Sarah Turpie
Senior project editor: Chris Marke
Marketing manager: Ruslana Khatagova
Cover design: Wendy Scott
Typeset by: C&M Digitals (P) Ltd, Chennai, India

Library of Congress Control Number: 2021944699

British Library Cataloguing in Publication Data

A catalogue record for this book is available from the British Library

ISBN 978-1-5297-5291-5
ISBN 978-1-5297-5290-8 (pbk)

Contents

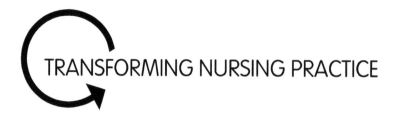

TRANSFORMING NURSING PRACTICE

Transforming Nursing Practice is a series tailor made for pre-registration student nurses. Each book addresses a core topic and is:

 Clearly written and easy to read

 Full of case studies and activities

✓ Mapped to the NMC Standards of proficiency for registered nurses

 Focused on applying theory to everyday nursing practice

Each book addresses a core topic and has been carefully developed to be simple to use, quick to read and written in clear language.

An invaluable series of books that explicitly relates to the NMC standards. Each book covers a different topic that students need to explore in order to develop into a qualified nurse... I would recommend this series to all Pre-Registered nursing students whatever their field or year of study.

LINDA ROBSON,
Senior Lecturer at Edge Hill University

Many titles in the series are on our recommended reading list and for good reason - the content is up to date and easy to read. These are the books that actually get used beyond training and into your nursing career.

EMMA LYDON,
Adult Student Nursing

ABOUT THE SERIES EDITORS

DR MOOI STANDING is an Independent Academic Nursing Consultant (UK and international) responsible for the core knowledge, personal and professional learning skills titles. She has invaluable experience as an NMC Quality Assurance Reviewer of educational programmes, and as a Professional Regulator Panellist on the NMC Practice Committee. Mooi is also a Board member of Special Olympics Malaysia.

DR SANDRA WALKER is a Clinical Academic in Mental Health working between North Bristol Trust and Southern Health Trust. She is series editor for the mental health nursing titles. She is a Qualified Mental Health Nurse with a wide range of clinical experience spanning 30 years and spent several years working as a mental health lecturer at Southampton University.

BESTSELLING TEXTBOOKS

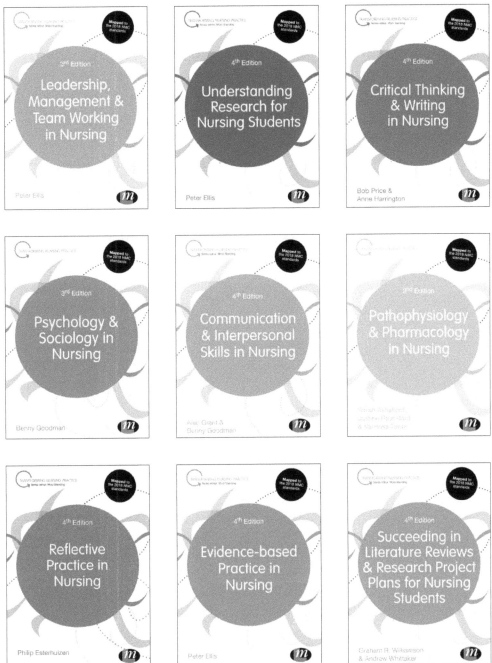

You can find a full list of textbooks in the *Transforming Nursing Practice* series at
uk.sagepub.com/TNP-series

Foreword

Delivering person-centred nursing care puts into words the excellent care nurses aspire to provide but often find difficult to explain. In developing and maintaining our professional identities as nurses, it is important that we can articulate, celebrate and emulate such good practice in caring for patients and other service users. If we are unable to do so, there is a danger that the knowledge or skills associated with high standards of person-centred nursing care remain hidden, not understood, or not used and valued as much as other approaches.

Building on the success of the first edition, the second edition of this excellent book has been thoughtfully updated and revised. The concept of person-centred nursing described stresses the importance of treating patients as individuals, and respecting their humanity. This requires nurses to elicit patients' narratives in order to understand: (i) their perceptions of the health problems they are experiencing; (ii) their hopes and fears in tackling problems; (iii) their expectations of health professionals and themselves regarding care interventions; and (iv) how to develop and refine ways of relating to patients in light of (i), (ii) and (iii). Stages of person-centred nursing care are described: anticipating, relating, negotiating, collaborating and evaluating. These are mapped against the nursing process to illustrate practical ways of integrating subjective person-centred values within objective, evidence-based, standardised systems of care. For example, relating, negotiating and collaborating augment assessment, planning and implementing respectively by engaging patients in meaningful partnership working, where possible, to identify and address their concerns and health needs. Four very detailed case studies demonstrate the successful application of person-centred skills in adult, learning disabilities, children and mental health nursing settings. It is recognised that patients can vary from passive recipients of care to proactive self-carers, and that some medical or environmental conditions are less conducive to person-centred care than others. A tension between limited resources and unlimited care demands is acknowledged, but it is argued that time invested in person-centred care can result in more successful rehabilitation and fewer remissions that would drain resources even further. It may also lead to greater patient satisfaction with healthcare services, and possibly more job satisfaction for nurses.

This book's cogent exploration and application of person-centred nursing knowledge and skills will be invaluable for readers wishing to develop their understanding and expertise in this area. It will help readers to achieve NMC standards of proficiency for registered nurses, for example: Platform 1: Being an accountable professional – providing nursing care that is person-centred, safe and compassionate (NMC, 2018, p7). It will also help readers to meet NMC Code requirements, for example: Prioritise people – 2: Listen to people and respond to their preferences and concerns (NMC, 2018, p6). I highly recommend this insightful book to all nursing students and to registered nurses negotiating NMC revalidation requirements.

Dr Mooi Standing, Series Editor

About the author

Bob Price is a healthcare education and training consultant. He started his clinical work as a nurse in trauma and then cancer care, developing new ways to address the altered body image needs of patients. Subsequently he led education programmes at the Royal Marsden Hospital (London), South Bank University, the RCN and the Open University. He has been a visiting lecturer to institutes within the UK, Europe and North America. Bob is also author of the SAGE text, *Critical Thinking and Writing in Nursing.*

Acknowledgements

No textbook comes from an author alone. There are editors and critical readers who offer wise counsel, so my sincere thanks to Laura Walmsley, Sarah Turpie and Mooi Standing and to the nurses with whom I explored case studies en route. The second edition of this textbook was written during the Covid-19 pandemic of 2020–21, something that reinforced to me the incredible lengths to which nurses have gone to humanise care, as well as saving many lives. Many nurses have been an inspiration for this book.

Introduction

Who is this book for?

This textbook is written for students learning how to nurse. But it will also be of value to registered nurses who are re-evaluating their work. The book is designed to help you to understand what person-centred care means, and how it can best operate alongside evidence-based care and promises made by the service (standard care packages and protocols). The book is about what you might do to deliver care in a person-centred way. Importantly, through case studies the book links the philosophy of person-centred care to the practicalities of delivering it in the clinical workplace. Case studies are drawn from across different fields of practice to illustrate the stages of person-centred care in action. Each case study includes a series of insights gained and practice tips for your guidance. Being person-centred is expressed differently as the care relationship develops. This second edition of this textbook has been written amidst the developing Covid-19 pandemic and its exceptional pressures upon healthcare services. The first case study (Chapter 3) is concerned with the rehabilitation of a patient recovering from this viral infection. The other three case studies reflect more optimistic times ahead, when care can once again diversify and become more tailored, benefiting from the protection afforded by vaccine programmes extending over the years to come.

In a time of pandemic it would be tempting to dismiss the idea that person-centred care is possible. However, this textbook argues that such care has always needed to remain pragmatic, reflecting the resources available. In pandemic times person-centred care may then centre much more on patients' fears, bolstering coping skills rather than necessarily extending choices. The concept of person-centred care remains important.

Why *Delivering Person-Centred Care?*

There are different recommendations about how you should practise and these tend to compete in their prescriptions for care. For example, evidence-based practice emphasises the need to deliver care that has been well researched and tested. It emphasises the need to deliver care that has a proven impact, especially in the area of treatments selected (Ellis, 2019). That which the nurse does or says should be based firmly upon science. But the nurse too is required to work effectively as a team member, to make good on the promises of the healthcare service. Here there is an emphasis on standard care, protocols and policies (Swanwick and Vaux, 2020). Much of this care agenda is driven by concerns for equity, ensuring that all service users have a reasonable share of resources. Equity isn't the same thing as equality. A patient combatting cancer will have greater needs than one perhaps having their gall bladder removed, so care is delivered proportionate to what we understand to be the challenges of different illnesses or injuries. In effect, standardised care packages assure the patient that they are not unfairly treated as regards promises made by the service. Against both of these 'should do' care recommendations, however, there is that which has most closely been associated with nursing care during the past decades. In the nursing models of care developed at the end of the 1900s nurses were encouraged to focus firmly upon the patient as a person, to discover needs and hopes that the individual had (Tripathy, 2019). The philosophy of nursing care has emphasised the negotiation of care, using a process of joint assessment, planning, action and evaluation that nurses know as the nursing process. This philosophy emphasises the tailoring of care wherever that is realistic.

The problem with so many recommendations about how care should be designed is that you might wonder: how do I manage my work in a way that meets everyone's expectations? How am I to know that I have practised professionally today? These are vitally important questions if you are to sustain a lifelong career in nursing. This usually entails clarifying what we mean by concepts in use (person-centred care) and then finding compromises with regard to meeting others' expectations of us. For example, a manager might insist that there is little scope to practise outside the standard offer of care, but you realise that a patient has pressing needs that must be met if that same offer is not to be undermined. You have to work within the system but retain the personal part of care as well. Research evidence might suggest the particular efficacy of a given treatment, but you have to relate the merits of that to the patient *and* understand what it entails for the patient to commit to the same. Modifications or adjustments might be necessary if the patient is to benefit from a treatment.

This book, then, is all about clarifying what person-centred care is and helping you to practise it in a way that both meets the needs of patients and others and enables you to affirm that you have acted professionally. It assists you to explore what person-centred care looks like at different stages in the nursing care process and helps you to deliberate on what seems practical there. Whilst many care recommendations describe an ideal, this book helps you understand the necessary compromises – that which seems realistic.

Book structure

The book is arranged in two parts. The first part describes the theory of person-centred care, whilst the second (Chapters 3–7) delivers a series of four patient case studies that exemplify person-centred care in action. Case studies are necessarily illustrations. They are not formulaic prescriptions for how all care must look, but by studying them you should quickly appreciate how concepts introduced in Part 1 of the book are actioned as part of nursing care. Case studies are drawn from each of the main divisions of nursing studies and reflect a range of patients or service users that you might meet. As you will see, however, case studies sometimes illustrate the need to consult with colleagues beyond a team. I would strongly recommend that you read all the case studies, irrespective of whether they reflect your division of nursing studies. Each case study has something to offer as regards turning ideas into action. The final chapter of Part 2 reflects on the case study insights and looks forward to the future. What have we really learned about person-centred care in action? What are the skill requirements if you are to enrich your care delivery in the future? I acknowledge that some changes may be necessary as regards the contracts of care that health services negotiate with the public.

We begin, though, with theory, in Part 1. In Chapter 1, I explain the concept of person-centred care and briefly how it has arisen as part of nursing philosophy. Person-centred care is not only important for improving care delivery; it has also been important in helping to define nursing. I set this account alongside other care recommendations, evidence-based care and standardised care, the better to help you understand the environment in which it has to operate.

In Chapter 2, I connect person-centred care to the nursing process. Nurses work back and forth in parallel, advancing an understanding of healthcare problems and challenges and building a working relationship with the patient. Without strategy, the nurse has little to offer the patient. Without a growing rapport with the patient as a person, the nurse has little chance of executing strategy in a way that is sustainable as well as effective. So in this chapter you will learn about the sequencing of care and the opportunities and challenges that arise there.

Requirements for the NMC *Standards of Proficiency for Registered Nurses*

The Nursing and Midwifery Council (NMC) has established standards of proficiency to be met by applicants to different parts of the register, and these are the standards it considers necessary for safe and effective practice. This book is structured so that it will help you to understand and meet the proficiencies required for entry to the NMC register. The relevant proficiencies are presented at the start of each chapter so that you can clearly see which ones the chapter addresses. The proficiencies have been designed to be generic so that they apply to all fields of nursing and all care settings. This is because all nurses must be able to meet the needs of any person they encounter in their practice, regardless of their stage of life or health challenges, whether these are mental, physical, cognitive or behavioural.

This book includes the latest standards for 2018 onwards, taken from *Future Nurse: Standards of Proficiency for Registered Nurses* (NMC, 2018).

Learning features

Learning by reading text is not always easy. Therefore, to provide variety and to assist with the development of independent learning skills and the application of theory to practice, this book contains activities, case studies, further reading, a glossary (p171) and useful websites to help you to manage your learning.

Some activities ask you to reflect on aspects of practice, or your experience of it, or the people or situations you encounter. *Reflection* is an essential skill in nursing, and it helps you to understand the world around you and often to identify how things might be improved. Other activities will help you develop key graduate skills, such as your ability to *think critically* about a topic in order to challenge received wisdom.

You might want to think about completing these activities as part of your personal development plan (PDP) or portfolio. After completing the activity, write it up in your PDP or portfolio in a section devoted to that particular skill, then look back over time to see how far you are developing. You can also do more of the activities for a key skill in which you have identified a weakness, which will help build your confidence in that area.

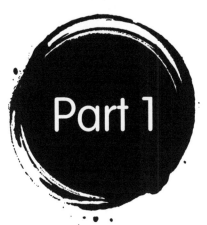

Part 1   Person-centred care

Theory and philosophy

Chapter 1 Person-centred care

Concepts, origins and challenges

NMC Future Nurse Standards of Proficiency for Registered Nurses

This chapter will address the following platforms and proficiencies:

Platform 1: Being an accountable professional
At the point of registration, the registered nurse will be able to:

1.8   demonstrate the knowledge, skills and ability to think critically when applying evidence and drawing on experience to make evidence-informed decisions in all situations.
1.9   understand the need to base all decisions regarding care and interventions on people's needs and preferences, recognising and addressing any personal and external factors that may unduly influence your decisions.
1.10   demonstrate resilience and emotional intelligence and be capable of explaining the rationale that influences your judgements and decisions in routine, complex and challenging situations.

Chapter aims

After reading this chapter, you will be able to:

- outline the origins of person-centred care within nursing and how it might be influenced by other recommendations for care;
- summarise why an understanding of partnership, role and patient expectations of care might all shape the form that person-centred care takes;
- reflect upon how key elements of person-centred care might by influenced by opportunities and challenges in your own chosen field of nursing practice.

Introduction

I want to start this chapter with the clinical context in which person-centred care operates. It is the context of care and competing care recommendations there that are at the heart of understanding both what person-centred care is and why it can be exciting but challenging to practise. You may already have appreciated that applying theory is not easy, so we start with commonly encountered difficulties and needs.

There are three recommended approaches to nursing care delivery and each of these is influential in the clinical environment. First (and central to this book), nurses have to relate successfully, sensitively and effectively with the patient and their family. As it is the person who experiences the injury, disability or illness and who determines what they will do in response to that, we must understand the person (Schellinger et al., 2018). If we are to persuade the patient to respond to health challenges in a beneficial way that also makes sense to them, then we had better work closely with their understanding, feelings, beliefs, values and aspirations. We have to be person-centred. We cannot simply instruct the patient to do what we believe is right. We must persuade them of what might be helpful and indeed arrive at that through exploration of what they feel that they need (King et al., 2019). We negotiate care, assess requirements together and plan strategies that will address needs and counter problems (Maloney et al., 2018). We action the care plan together; some things will be contributed by the nurse and some by the patient or family. Later we jointly evaluate how the care has proceeded. This is the essence of person-centred care.

Two other nursing care approaches compete for your attention. The first of these is evidence-based practice. This approach to nursing care recommends that we direct our work based upon evidence drawn from research and other rigorously arranged means of gathering and collating information (e.g. patient surveys, care audits) (Jolley, 2020). It is argued that the nurse works as a scientist, researching what is important in healthcare – that experienced by patients with the same diagnosis, for example. We focus upon how treatments work and which of them have the widest and longest-lasting beneficial effect. In evidence-based practice it is argued that some knowledge is superior to other knowledge, and that we should trust it more because of the way it was gathered and analysed. This puts a rather different slant on the approach to care because the nurse is often cast as the expert who recommends particular courses of action because of what research has revealed. In evidence-based care the emphasis shifts from patient choice and towards knowledge and its expert application.

The third recommended approach to nursing care comes from a variety of sources, from organisations such as the National Institute for Health and Care Excellence (NICE) (www.nice.org.uk), and from employers and care forums where expert practice has been reviewed and research evidence may have been distilled. Such organisations create a range of standards, protocols and policies that direct how healthcare teams should work and what provision should be made for patients. Protocols are driven by research, but they are informed too by that which is judged value for money (healthcare resources are finite). In the midst of a pandemic, for example, there is a rapid identification and sharing of best-treatment protocols – that which rescues extremely ill patients. Rather loosely, we might call this approach standardised care, with packages of provision that reassure the public what the healthcare organisation will provide and against which provision can be judged. Whilst care packages might take different and sometimes innovative forms, Sekhon et al. (2017) have highlighted the challenges of weaving client acceptability into the design of healthcare provision. You may have met elements of standardised care upon joining a clinical placement, through care protocols, policies and perhaps standard care packages associated with particular treatments. If in person-centred care the emphasis is upon the person and care negotiated, then in standardised care the emphasis is upon transparent and consistent service to a population of patients. Standardised care sets parameters on what care is counted as desirable, safe and within service constraints.

Activity 1.1   Reflection

Review now any recent experience of clinical placements and decide whether Table 1.1 helps explain some of the learning challenges that you encountered there. Were there instances where different nursing care recommendations seemed to clash with each other, where guidance on what you *should do* clashed with what it seemed possible to do?

An outline answer is given at the end of this chapter.

Table 1.1   Approaches to nursing care delivery

Recommended care approach	Short description	Practical implications
Person-centred care	Care that is arranged through a careful analysis of patient experiences and needs, working closely with their coping and preferred objectives. Care is conceived strongly in terms of partnership and the adoption of mutually beneficial roles that advance the jointly agreed plan of care.	In an ideal world person-centred care is tailor-made, entirely focused upon the unique needs of the individual, but cognisant of what research and other sources of evidence has to offer. Care is negotiated, jointly reviewed and updated, implying the availability of significant nursing skills and resources in time and material (McCormack and McCance, 2017).

(Continued)

Table 1.1   (Continued)

Recommended care approach	Short description	Practical implications
Evidence-based care	Care draws critically and consistently upon the growing body of research evidence relating to illness, treatment, therapy and care, and upon research insights into patient coping and motivation. There is a significant emphasis upon nursing as a science – that which examines and utilises the best information available.	Evidence frequently focuses upon that which applies to the many, and that which is more predictive or insightful as regards what happens or is required in healthcare. Powerful evidence is often that which is believed to predict what might happen next, in terms of risk, improvement or deterioration, and that which works consistently (Heaslip and Bruce, 2019). We might then prescribe treatment or care measures on the basis of evidence rather than individual patient capacity or readiness to engage.
Standardised care	Standardised care focuses upon promising the wider population quality-assured treatment and care measures that the healthcare organisation has committed to and which helps to ensure that finite resources are equitably shared, based on an understanding of the challenges posed by different diagnoses. It is typically expressed in treatment protocols – that which healthcare teams commit to and may later be measured by.	This approach offers the nurse reassurance about what is sanctioned by the healthcare organisation. However, standardised care can seem inflexible and bureaucratic. Whilst it helps to cement a multidisciplinary approach to healthcare (all understand what the others are delivering), it admits only limited adjustment to care planning. The care package feels like exactly that: a package, transparent but relatively rigid.

Some of the problems with learning to nurse are associated with translating the different approaches to nursing care into action. Few would pretend that the nurse can afford to entirely tailor-make care with an individual patient (other patients compete for the nurse's attention). There are system, ethical, financial and skill constraints associated with that (Price, 2020). Nurses are, though, unlikely to espouse rigid care that takes little account of the individual patient. Whilst nurses wish to practise in an evidence-based way, that which is proven to be valuable and safe, evidence can be incomplete or contradictory and it can be complex to translate into daily care (Renolen et al., 2018). In effect, then, the three approaches to nursing care set checks and balances upon one another. Person-centred care reminds us that patients are people rather than subjects of a bureaucratic system. Evidence-based care reminds us that the nurse should not embark upon flights of fancy when planning care with patients. Standardised care reminds us that we contribute to a healthcare team and through that a service. What we negotiate with the patient often involves conferring with others and referring patients to other resources. The care has to be both realistic and joined up.

Key features of person-centred care

We turn now to what person-centred care is. You might infer from the above that I think it is something used judiciously, in a way that works with the other approaches to care outlined above. Byrne et al. (2020) observe that person-centred care is extremely hard to define, and this is because it has been used to serve different purposes. So, for example, person-centred care can be used to help define nursing and to distinguish it from other professions such as medicine. Person-centred care is polemical, a political discourse on how nursing should be (see, for example, McCormack and McCance, 2017). But person-centred care can also be extremely pragmatic. It can begin from another place where it is observed that patients make very personal decisions about what counts as an illness or problem and decide what they will then do about that (e.g. Brokerhof et al., 2020). No matter what diseases or injuries are diagnosed, patients can and do manage both health and illness in very individual ways. If we don't attend to that, working with their perceptions, definition of events and goals, then we are less likely to care for them successfully. Table 1.2 summarises some of the origins of person-centred nursing care today and notes how such origins have shaped descriptions of the approach.

Table 1.2   Origins of person-centred nursing care

Origin	Notes
Nursing and its professional credentials	For over a century, nurses have fought to detail what characterises their professional practice and to distinguish it in particular from medicine (Meleis, 2018). If nursing was more than an adjunct to medicine, then it became necessary to understand what constituted care. Two key tenets were that care was methodical (arranged in a nursing process) and that it centred firmly upon understanding the person who suffered a healthcare problem or disability. Nurses did not simply counter diseases and injuries.

(Continued)

Table 1.2   (Continued)

Origin	Notes
Nursing models of care	In the second half of the 20th century a series of different models were created that conceptualised care (McKenna et al., 2014). These often focused heavily upon the care relationship. Orem, for example, described nursing care as something that supplemented self-care – what the patient could do for themselves (Orem et al., 2003). In such models there was a strong emphasis on partnering patients, something that person-centred care also emphasises.
Holism	Holism is the philosophy that we best understand human beings from a full appreciation of their different dimensions. People are physical, psychological, social and spiritual (Donnelly, 2012). It was therefore not adequate to simply manage a problem in one dimension; treating a wound, for example. The clinician had to understand how the wound made the patient feel; how it might impact on their daily living. Holism as a philosophy is not unique to nursing, but it has mandated enquiry into the patient's experiences and need. We need to understand how an illness, injury or disability fits into the individual's world.
Discourses on patient compliance, self-care and successful longer-term management.	There has been growing social and psychology evidence relating to how patients make use of healthcare guidance and treatment (e.g. consumerism) (Latimer et al., 2017; Marx and Padmanabhan, 2021). In some instances patients have failed to heed the advice offered and may even have continued with lifestyles likely to damage their health. Attention has therefore focused increasingly upon how patients interpret risks, needs and goals and how they evaluate and utilise healthcare services. An appreciation of health beliefs and values has challenged clinicians to work more closely with the patient's own perceptions.

In this book person-centred care is defined as a judicious approach used by the nurse to help patients and their relatives make the most meaningful use of the healthcare services available to them. It centres upon the patient as a person, someone who interprets their own healthcare circumstances and who tries to fit illness, injury or disability (health changes) into what it means to lead a meaningful life. Person-centred care describes the way in which the nurse offers a partnership to the patient, respecting what the patient believes confronts them and then helping them to make plans that counter the problems identified. Person-centred care alerts the patient to relevant evidence about what might be helpful and it honestly acquaints the individual with what is available through healthcare services. Person-centred care describes a professional and supportive relationship that enacts and reviews jointly agreed care measures and which evaluates progress thereafter.

People, practice and power

Byrne et al. (2020), in their literature review, describe person-centred care as premising things about people, practice and power. People are understood as regards their uniqueness – the very individual way in which they live and manage their health or illness. There is an emphasis upon partnering the patient in the business of under-standing and managing changed health circumstances. Put bluntly, nurses don't tell the patient what to do.

Practice involves the adoption of roles – those that are mutually beneficial and which demonstrate the nurse's empathetic interest in the patient. The partners in care decide who does what and how those contributions relate to one another. Practice also involves what Byrne et al. (2020) call space. The patient has the right to choose what to do. They can give or withhold consent to treatment, but more than that, they commit effort and energy to varying degrees to work that has been judged as important to treat-ment, recovery or rehabilitation. With such space comes responsibility. The patient is jointly responsible for care outcomes, at least where they have committed to make con-tributions of their own.

Power is expressed with regard to patients choosing care options with the nurse (they share planning), but it also refers to the need for nurses to sometimes advocate patient needs within a healthcare system that might not always recognise personal needs or care opportunities.

Concerning the person

Let's look more closely at the person and what this care approach presumes there.

Activity 1.2   Critical thinking

Consider now the following statements, which are implicit in getting to know a patient as a person, and which help build a working rapport with them. Speculate why you think each is important and what limits there might be to the same. As you think about this, base your thoughts on your own field of nursing. What make these essential or problematic in mental health, child health, learning disability needs or adult nursing, for example? Then read on to review my reasoning.

1. Patients start as strangers, so we have to anticipate possible concerns, interests and needs before they arrive. We have (as it were) to cue ourselves in to likely worries and needs – that which upon subsequent meeting assures them that we are concerned for their wellbeing.
2. Patients vary in the extent to which they permit nurse enquiry, evaluating what seems necessary to enable them to secure desired assistance. Some patients are more private than others.
3. People attend as much to their symptoms as any signs of illness or injury. If we are to establish a rapport, then we must pay attention to both. If we are to successfully know the person, then we must start with their experiences.

As this answer is based on your own reflection, there is no outline answer at the end of this chapter.

It may have surprised you that I think person-centred care starts before you even meet the patient. It begins with identifying the more common concerns, difficulties and challenges that patients experience when they come into your care. So, for example, in mental healthcare the nurse had better begin with an already working appreciation of what it feels like to experience hallucinations and delusions before they start to personalise care for a patient suffering from psychosis (Price, 2016; Ratcliffe, 2017). In child health nursing the nurse has to anticipate how children might conceive of pain before a problem can be confirmed (Pate et al., 2019). The cataloguing of commonly occurring worries and needs, met by patients, in your own field of nursing cues you into how questions might be directed during history taking. The emphasis on what *might* worry the individual patient increases the likelihood that they find your enquiries knowledgeable, empathetic and reassuring. This has significant implications for nurses working in clinical specialisms. They need to remain up to date, reading about relevant worries and needs as well as developments associated with treatments. For you as a student, this has implications when going on clinical placement. It is important for you to conduct some preparatory reading about recurrent patient concerns and needs in that area of practice.

To anticipate possible patient concerns and anxieties is not to assume that all patients experience the same things. Human beings vary markedly in their past experience of illness and their confidence in dealing with change (Heffer and Willoughby, 2017). We are not requiring patients to fit a formula of care requirements. We do, however, need to manage the number of questions that we pose when taking a patient history. We are not interrogating the patient. By starting with questions that are more likely to be of concern to the patient, however, we might encourage report of their experiences. It is important to ask open questions – those that are not easily answered with yes or no. So, for example, 'Can you describe how this has felt these last few days?' not only invites a recounting of experiences but might also signal what constitutes 'the problem' for the patient.

Much of person-centred care is predicated upon a patient's willingness to open up to the nurse's enquiries, to reveal what the problem means to them (Riding et al., 2017). Your own clinical experience to date may already have revealed that some patients are more private than others. Some assume that doctors and nurses confine themselves to discrete areas, such as altered body function, or the presence or otherwise of pain. Patients come from different cultures and have different expectations of how the nurse should behave (Galanti, 2015). In some cultures, for example, it is the head of the household who responds to the nurse's questions. If you are studying child health nursing, you may have already observed that children can be very circumspect about revealing their concerns to you. The readiness and ability of patients to reveal more about themselves varies markedly and liaison with the parent becomes vital. In child health nursing, person-centred care is expressed as family-centred care for that reason (Dennis et al., 2017). A patient with a learning difficulty may struggle to represent their experiences and feelings. These are important points because what the patient sometimes conceives of as coping might be part of the problem. Abuse of alcohol or drugs, for instance, might be a coping mechanism, but unless the nurse can help the patient profile the problem, then care is more difficult to negotiate (Linden-Carmichael et al., 2019).

In person-centred care the nurse has to develop skills in enabling the patient to reveal more about their perceptions of the problem – what represents coping and progress to them and what might sustain them in recovery or rehabilitation. The nurse will not necessarily become a psychotherapist, but they must strive to be a confidant. This is especially important when patients deal with chronic illnesses and must learn to manage their own treatment (Russell et al., 2019). However, clinical settings then profoundly affect the extent to which the nurse can advance an understanding of the patient. In the casualty department, for example, there is usually scant time to explore coping (Noble et al., 2019). Instead, the nurse is focused more upon risk and its management. In chronic illness care, in many mental health settings and in palliative care the opportunities to know and understand the patient are clearly greater. If you start with a rather idealised notion of person-centred care, one in which the patient quickly reveals everything of concern, you may be disappointed. In reality, some patients may only reveal a very limited amount about their selves and negotiate a more superficial partnership with you (Launer, 2018). Nonetheless, where you respect that preference, they may still evaluate the care as excellent.

I would encourage you to focus just as much on the patient's symptoms as on any signs or tests that might attend the opening of the care relationship. Signs and tests are dispassionate and they seem like the realm of the medical rather than the personal problem. Symptoms seem rather more the realm of the person and for a very good reason. The ways in which patients describe their symptoms are very individual and they enable the nurse to access the narrative that the patient runs concerning what is needed (Launer, 2018). When human beings face an illness or confront an injury, they develop a storyline (a narrative) to explain the matter to themselves and indeed any trusted listener. The person-centred care nurse wishes to understand that narrative. For example, a patient typically describes how the problem felt (perhaps as a type of pain), the context of it happening (when it came on and how long it lasted), what they thought was wrong ('goodness, I thought it was cancer') and what they then did about it. A great deal can be learned from patients as you listen to their symptoms and encourage them to extend that into an account of experiences. So, person-centred care accesses the person through signs and symptoms and, beyond that, through narratives.

Patient narrative is defined in this book as the way in which the individual accounts for their experience of illness, injury or health difficulty, and that which may shape their attitudes and values regarding what it means to cope and to accept or reject assistance. The patient narrative is not necessarily rational; it might be based on folk beliefs and it could form a defence against change. The narrative of an individual who persists with cigarette smoking despite respiratory problems, for example, is every bit as important to understand as one that demonstrates insight into risk. Patient narratives can have a profound effect on how patients interpret healthcare. We can only understand the patient narrative through sensitive questioning and the building of a trusting and supportive care relationship. Through such questions patients sometimes uncover a previously unrecognised and unspoken narrative, one relating to deeply felt attitudes and values. So learning about a narrative can sometimes be challenging for the patient and nurse alike.

Activity 1.3   Critical thinking

Jot down what you think the implications of a patient narrative might be for nursing care. Have you used a narrative to make sense of a health change that you have experienced? Have you listened to others' narratives outside of the hospital, for example a child describing their worries about going to school?

An outline answer is given at the end of this chapter.

Concerning practice

At one level, person-centred care sounds as though the nurse is simply nice. It would be easy to suggest that the concept is an overly complex way of saying be polite towards patients. Person-centred care, though, involves rather more than that. It involves not only considerate communication, but partnership and collaborative work as well (Backman et al., 2019). When you first thought about becoming a nurse you might have anticipated all the things that you would do for the patient. That would seem especially fulfilling when patients are incapacitated and when they necessarily rely on what others provide. For example, a patient in Covid-19 respiratory distress requires comprehensive care. This is nursing as traditionally conceived as service, a vocation to care for the incapacitated. Person-centred care, however, presumes that in a majority of cases, when the patient is conscious and able to provide at least some self-care, collaboration and shared planning will be the order of the day.

It is worth pausing to consider the significance of this. What does partnering in care entail? What will it mean to engage the patient in joint planning of care measures, those that draw heavily upon the patient's experiences and perceived needs? The first thing it entails is the building of a professional working rapport (Senteio and Yoon, 2020). Patients need to feel that they can trust you and that requires you to demonstrate an obvious concern for their continued wellbeing. Understanding the patient and how they feel is not limited to first assessment. You will need to signal an enthusiastic interest in how they experience your care too. The next thing that it involves is the development of collaborative roles that the nurse and the patient fulfil. Table 1.3 indicates some of the roles that may be used in a person-centred care relationship.

Table 1.3 Possible person-centred care roles

Role	Notes
Problem analyst	In some instances patients come to care without a clear diagnosis and then the nature of a healthcare problem has to be analysed. Both patient and nurse may bring expertise to the problem analysis, the patient, for instance, reviewing how they typically think of problems, approach risks and motivate themselves. Problem analysis has a large part to play in mental health nursing and it can be important too in children's care as nurse, child and parent analyse the difficulties faced.
Advisor-counsellor	Nurses frequently function as advisors to patients; indeed, this role is critical when patients determine what course of action they will follow. It is important, though, to note that the advisory role extends towards counselling only to the extent of the nurse's advance skills education. Person-centred care does not assume that all nurses are psychotherapists, with the skill, confidence and education to equip them to guide patients through difficult personal insights. Quite frequently person-centred care nurses utilise their experience of what past patients have found useful to better advise a new patient. Nurses are uniquely well placed to explain the different ways in which patients have previously tackled challenges.
Listener	Person-centred care nurses listen to strategic purpose. Everything that the patient feels able to share signals something about their current state, confidence and progress. At the heart of person-centred care is the argument that perceptions are as powerful as facts. The nurse works with the patient's perceptions the better to address problems and advance towards agreed goals.
Teacher or coach	Nurses explain a great deal (e.g. about treatment, grief reactions, stages of rehabilitation) and this quickly becomes teaching or coaching. Of course, where there are teachers or coaches, there are learners, and learning is especially important where a patient tackles a chronic illness. Some advanced practice roles major in teaching and coaching patients using the specialist knowledge of the nurse. Sometimes, however, patients teach nurses, especially where the patient is accomplished in coping strategies (e.g. managing diabetes).
Critical reviewer	The nurse might be asked to review progress with the patient, to explore doubts about the direction of rehabilitation or the patient's confidence in self-care. The nurse will need to be both empathetic and honest as progress is reviewed.
Strategist	Both patients and nurses might act as strategists, anticipating the challenges ahead and what might work best. At the start of the care relationship it is often the nurse that is the strategist because of their greater knowledge of care facilities. Later, however, strategy leadership is likely to be shared and even to shift towards the patient as the problems are better understood.
Consultant	Here consultant is used in the sense of someone who introduces the individual to resources and opportunities; who helps the patient to realise possibilities. Expert nurses are aware of a wide range of resources that patients might tap into.

In the next chapter we will be exploring the relationship between person-centred care and the nursing process. Suffice to say here, however, that the practice relationship with the patient is a dynamic one. What might start with the nurse leading a great deal, and perhaps providing a majority of the care, gradually becomes a relationship where the patient expresses much more of their own coping and self-care skills, making decisions that fit their personal circumstances. That this is both morally and economically important is perhaps evident. In chronic illness, for example, there are insufficient resources for all care to be delivered by the nurse. In any case, patients build self-esteem and confidence from shouldering incrementally greater amounts of care responsibility.

Concerning power

Person-centred care is committed to empowering patients, enabling them to take charge of their personal healthcare circumstances and to represent their needs to service providers (McCormack and McCance, 2017). The basis for this is informed consent (the moral and legal right of most patients to determine what happens to their body) and then, too, an empathetic commitment to helping patients to live well. In many cases an illness or injury cannot be entirely corrected. The patient must manage residual problems whilst hopefully sustaining a good quality of life. Successful nursing care is then not about the patient necessarily becoming better, but about them feeling whole, dignified and purposeful again.

Activity 1.4   Critical thinking

Jot down now some of the circumstances that you already know about when it is unrealistic for patients to give entirely informed consent to suggested treatment and care measures. What do you think this means for the delivery of person-centred care?

An outline answer is given at the end of this chapter.

Whilst the goal of patient empowerment has featured quite strongly within person-centred care, rather less has been discussed as regards its practical implications (Ocloo and Matthews, 2015). It is assumed, for example, that the patient wishes to be empowered; to take charge of a share of the care decision making. In some situations a patient might observe that such empowerment involves offloading the responsibilities of care onto themself or their family. Patients or lay carers may protest that they do not have the skills or the resources to shoulder a greater responsibility for care. In these circumstances person-centred care finds itself at the uncomfortable junction between patient advocacy (representing the patient's needs) and acknowledgement of service limitations. Healthcare resources are limited; the provision has to be shared amongst multiple patients with pressing demands. In some instances the patient might be referred to other care agencies that can support them (e.g. charities, self-help support groups) and encouraged to explore different ways in which felt needs can be met. However, the uncomfortable fact remains that if the patient and family cannot achieve a greater degree of self-care, then some future deficits and problems may arise. Such frank analysis might surprise you in a book about person-centred care. However, the nurse has only so much to offer the patient. That such care is articulated well, adjusted as far as possible to meet individual care needs, is central to the ethos of person-centred care. It remains a fact, however, that you will be unable to address every felt need of the patient.

Central to the power component of person-centred care is the concept of dignity (Zirak et al., 2017). The nurse works both to protect the dignity of the person and to promote it through the discovery of what the patient can achieve. This is one of the reasons why nurses so often act as advisors, teachers and coaches when practising person-centred care. The nurse teaches the patient, illustrating what might be attempted. Nurses have a responsibility under the NMC code of conduct (NMC, 2018) to alert their superiors and, if necessary, the NMC itself to deficits in care provision that threaten the integrity and wellbeing of the patient. Where patients are left unattended in parlous condition, it is both the professional and the person-centred care responsibility of the nurse to alert their superiors to deficits in care and to record their concerns. This is important in person-centred care because the nurse cannot build an effective relationship with the patient unless trust is established. The patient must know that if they raise reasonable concerns with the nurse, this will be adequately represented to those in charge of resources and policy in that area.

The person-centred care environment

To practise in a person-centred way is synonymous with helping patients (Doherty and Thompson, 2014; Sharp et al., 2016). You may already have realised, however, that if the environment surrounding the nurse does not also espouse person-centred care, then difficulties will arise. Juggling the three different care approaches requires judgement and support from colleagues and superiors.

McCormack and McCance (2017) observe that for person-centred care to advance, four things must be firmly in place:

1. Nurses must be emotionally and skill-competent. They must have the necessary interpersonal skills, commitment, and clarity of beliefs and values associated with what seems most desirable in care activity. Table 1.3, for example, suggests a number of roles that make skill demands upon the nurse.

2. There must be a conducive care environment – one that accepts the necessity of shared decision making between clinicians and patients. There are significant implications here for the resourcing of the health service and role responsibilities when risk is assessed.

3. There must be person-centred care processes in place – the means by which agreed care can be planned and documented. The Gothenburg University Centre for Person-centred Care commissioned a series of studies exploring what was involved in delivering person-centred care (Brittan et al., 2016). While there were similarities as regards the ethos of care, local practical measures were needed to accommodate the different care environments.

4. Expected outcomes have to be better explained. There are multiple ways in which person-centred care might be evaluated, for example in terms of expressed patient satisfaction, success in rehabilitation programmes, statistical improvements in body functions and exercise tolerance. Without being clear about what is a claimed result of person-centred care, it is harder to persuade others to adopt it.

Significantly, modern healthcare organisations increasingly involve members of the public and often patients in their clinical governance systems. Public governors contribute to the running of healthcare organisations and the strategies they develop to improve services. It is recognised that if organisations are to reduce the risk of complaints, there is an advantage in engaging patients in shared decision making in the first instance. When we evaluate progress in a jointly negotiated plan of care, we assess what has been achieved by patient, nurse, and others in partnership. The success of this, however, depends upon a clear and well-articulated plan of action and that involves the nurse in revisiting the nursing process. It is to this that we turn in the next chapter.

Activity 1.5 Reflection

Think now of a recent clinical placement that you have completed or indeed a healthcare organisation that you have received service from either as a patient or a relative. What about that organisation seemed especially person-centred? What seemed more difficult to personalise in their provision?

An outline answer is given at the end of this chapter.

Chapter summary

This chapter started by exploring the complexity of clinical practice, where different recommendations compete for the guidance of your nursing care work. Person-centred care, evidence-based care and standardised care are not entirely mutually exclusive – each emphasises something of merit within healthcare – but different care approaches do help explain why clinical practice and learning can seem rather confusing. Each of the approaches raises checks and balances on the others, requiring the nurse to think carefully about how they proceed. Having started from that commonly encountered experience, the chapter offered a definition of person-centred care and encouraged you to review what that entails with regard to the person, to practice and to power within nursing care. The origins of person-centred care help to shape how different writers discuss the concept, but what remains central to the approach is a professional regard for the individual patient's experiences, perceptions and needs, and their right to negotiate care with the nurse and others who provide healthcare services. That negotiation is mediated by a variety of factors: the roles that nurses and patients might play, the level of intrusion that seems tolerable to the patient, and the practical resources and limitations that might be associated with a given care environment.

Activities: Brief outline answers

Activity 1.1 Reflection (p9)

In my experience, standardised care can dominate reasoning within clinical practice, in part because managers are hard-pressed to allocate precious resources and in part because patients and families have become increasingly discerning 'consumers' of healthcare services. Arranging care so as to minimise the risk of complaint can come to dominate the healthcare agenda. Culturally we think of healthcare as a service, detailing what is done for us, rather than what we collaborate upon, making contributions of our own as patients. Public health (that which prevents or limits illness) has been conceived elsewhere well away from the hospital environment. This means that for person-centred care to thrive, not only must we persuade colleagues to invest in it, but we must also convince patients and families that there are material benefits in collaborating on care.

Beyond this, it can be taxing to weave evidence into shared care planning with a patient. One of the reasons for this is that evidence is sometimes fragmented or contradictory. There is much more evidence available as regards treatments than there is about the psychology of illness, coping and recovery. In consequence, the nurse has to imagine how evidence of a more medical kind might be introduced to the patient as personally advantageous. The evidence has not only to be robust but utilisable as well. For that reason, the nurse often uses evidence to suggest ways to narrow down options when debating future plans with the patient.

Activity 1.3 Critical thinking (p16)

I wonder if you noted that patient narratives can complicate what seems acceptable care and what then is counted as a successful care relationship. You see, if the patient narrative is powerful, framing how the patient negotiates care with the nurse, it can become a limiting factor on what is achievable. A patient open to sharing their narrative and perhaps modifying it may achieve more than a patient who is resistant to all change. One of the challenges of person-centred care is to help the patient tell their story. This forms the basis of our assessment of what patients then already know and what they believe coping to consist of. That can raise some difficulties, for example if we have to gently refute their understanding of an illness, or of a risk such as obesity or cigarette smoking.

Other places where you may have heard narratives in use often centre on where something has gone wrong. Narratives are, for instance, exercised around marital divorce, or when an individual fails to secure a promotion or is made redundant. But narratives can explain success as well – for instance, the 'self-made individual'. Success is not simply about luck! Our first reaction towards narratives may be to see them as excuses, perhaps as distortions of reality, but in fact human beings routinely story their lives, making it possible to discern what counts as progress, good fortune or a critical period in their life.

Nurses routinely ask about signs, symptoms and problems, but the person-centred nurse asks about how the individual explains these issues to themselves and how that then shapes how they respond. It is from this unique beginning that the nurse can then negotiate care that seems tailor-made. The person-centred nurse helps the patient see the fit offered by care measures to their individual needs. The person-centred care nurse helps the patient understand how they can use, adapt or develop available resources.

Activity 1.4 Critical thinking (p18)

Your answers here may be closely associated with your own field of nursing. So, for example, if you work with clients who have difficulties learning, understanding complex healthcare information can be difficult. Information may have to be delivered in smaller chunks and understanding checked at each stage before you can ascertain that consent is informed and care can advance. It is clearly impossible for an unconscious patient to give informed consent to care, whilst in child health nursing the child's level of reasoning development might not be equal to the treatment decisions that have to be jointly made. In such circumstances a family member might have to assist in the negotiation of care. Beyond these examples you may have noted that person-centred care faces difficulties too when the patient's reasoning ability varies over time, for example associated with dementia.

Activity 1.5 Reflection (p20)

My example comes from hospice care and visits made to a dying relative there. Hospices have an excellent reputation for delivering very individual care. I stopped to consider what it was about the care approach that seemed especially good. I noted two things:

1. How much the nurses knew about how my relative fitted the illness to living, and her preferred daily activities. They knew what my relative liked to do and how the illness interrupted that.

2. The way the nurses interpreted therapy – in this case, the available analgesia regimen. My relative valued alertness over comfort; she defined herself through her ability to reason. Too much analgesia interrupted that, making her sleepy, so she preferred to tolerate some pain as a trade-off. The nurses then used non-pharmacological measures (physiotherapy and massage) to counter the residual pain.

Further reading

Buetow, S (2016) *Person-Centred Health Care: Balancing the Welfare of Clinicians and Patients.* London: Routledge.

Reading the more philosophical/polemical texts on person-centred care, you might wonder just what it takes for the clinician to meet all of the possible expectations of some patients. Consumerism and person-centred care could combine to fuel a relentless series of demands upon the resources, skills and knowledge of the practitioner. Buetow, though, searches for a balance between clinician and patient welfare that I think is refreshing. Person-centred care is about protecting humanity within care, and that extends to the endeavours of healthcare professionals as well as patients and their families.

Tees, S (ed.) (2016) *Person-Centred Approaches in Healthcare: A Handbook for Nurses and Midwives.* London: Open University Press.

One of the problems with most person-centred care textbooks is that they are relatively theoretical. There is a paucity of practice application. Not so this text, which compiles contributions from different chapter authors, illustrating using vignettes how care philosophy is expressed in a range of settings. Examples of care in action are necessarily selective (as in my own volume) – not everything can be illustrated – but there is a range of thoughtful discussion available.

Useful websites

What person-centred care means: RCNI 2017 (access through **www.rcni.com** and search 'what person-centred care means').

This feature, which extends to 91 pages of down-to-earth explanation, sets person-centred care in the context of the role of the healthcare assistant. The explanation is contextualised against healthcare settings as potentially dangerous, imposing and alien environments into which patients come. It emphasises the clinician's role in protecting the rights of patients and advancing their role in deciding how health problems are investigated and tackled. At base, person-centred care exemplifies what patient informed consent entails and it begins with an understanding of why patients may feel or be vulnerable.

Chapter 2 Person-centred care and the nursing process

NMC Future Nurse Standards of Proficiency for Registered Nurses

This chapter will address the following platforms and proficiencies:

Platform 1: Being an accountable professional

At the point of registration, the registered nurse will be able to:

1.10 demonstrate resilience and emotional intelligence and be capable of explaining the rationale that influences your judgements and decisions in routine, complex and challenging situations.

1.18 demonstrate the knowledge and confidence to contribute effectively and proactively in an interdisciplinary team.

Platform 4: Providing and evaluating care

At the point of registration, the registered nurse will be able to:

4.1 demonstrate and apply an understanding of what is important to people and how to use this knowledge to ensure their needs for safety, dignity, privacy, comfort and sleep can be met, acting as a role model for others in providing evidence-based person-centred care.

4.2 work in partnership with people to encourage shared decision-making, in order to support individuals, their families and carers to manage their own care when appropriate.

Chapter aims

After reading this chapter, you will be able to:

- relate person-centred care to the developing stages of the nursing process;
- describe how building a practical, collaborative and respectful relationship with the patient enables you to demonstrate personalised care.

Introduction

In the last chapter we explored the key features of person-centred care, relating it immediately to the problem of arranging nursing care in an environment that also commends evidence-based practice and where standard care packages assure the patient about the service provided. We now explore how person-centred care is enacted and compare that to the stages of the nursing process. This is an important consideration as person-centred care is expressed as an explorative care relationship, whilst the nursing process describes our work in terms of a methodical approach to problem solving. In person-centred care the problem is not an abstract or separate matter; it is something understood through the patient (Buckley et al., 2018). Person-centred care emphasises exploration, something that may be hampered by time constraints and strict stages. When I discuss this with students they usually observe that care has to progress through the nursing process faster than seems possible within person-centred care. If you are going to learn to nurse with confidence, though, you are going to have to marry the two – relationship building and problem solving.

It is tempting to think about person-centred care in idealistic terms. We wish to show how unique nursing work is. But as indicated in Chapter 1, person-centred care has to work pragmatically. We need to advance the care relationship sensitively but relatively quickly, at least in acute-care environments (Price, 2017). We work with what the patient feels comfortable with, that which they will permit relating to care enquiry and, later, role sharing, but this cannot be entirely at the expense of care commitments to others.

Two processes

Whilst the nursing process proceeds through four stages (assessing, planning, implementing and evaluating), person-centred care proceeds through five stages (anticipating, relating, negotiating, collaborating and evaluating). Figure 2.1 illustrates how the two processes parallel one another.

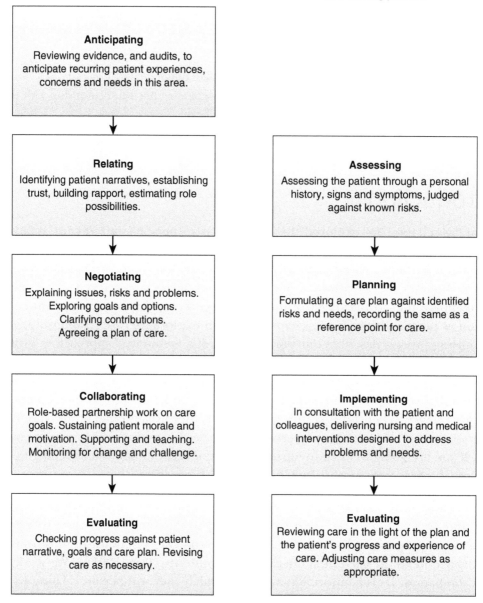

Person-centred care

The nursing process

Anticipating
Reviewing evidence, and audits, to anticipate recurring patient experiences, concerns and needs in this area.

Relating
Identifying patient narratives, establishing trust, building rapport, estimating role possibilities.

Assessing
Assessing the patient through a personal history, signs and symptoms, judged against known risks.

Negotiating
Explaining issues, risks and problems. Exploring goals and options. Clarifying contributions. Agreeing a plan of care.

Planning
Formulating a care plan against identified risks and needs, recording the same as a reference point for care.

Collaborating
Role-based partnership work on care goals. Sustaining patient morale and motivation. Supporting and teaching. Monitoring for change and challenge.

Implementing
In consultation with the patient and colleagues, delivering nursing and medical interventions designed to address problems and needs.

Evaluating
Checking progress against patient narrative, goals and care plan. Revising care as necessary.

Evaluating
Reviewing care in the light of the plan and the patient's progress and experience of care. Adjusting care measures as appropriate.

Figure 2.1   Person-centred care and the nursing process

Activity 2.1   Critical thinking

Study Figure 2.1 now to identify what you think are the chief differences between the stages of person-centred care and the nursing process. Both are methodical, one has five stages and one four, but what beyond that seems different about the two? Once you have noted some ideas, read on to my discussion below.

As this answer is based on your own reflection, there is no outline answer at the end of the chapter.

I wonder if you spotted that person-centred care is mediated very strongly through the care relationship and an understanding of patient experiences, perceptions and needs? This is not to argue that the nursing process has no regard for the patient as a person – on the contrary, it does – but in person-centred care the nurse tries to see illness, problems and solutions through the patient's eyes (Naldemirci et al., 2020). It is accepted that illness is understood through patient experience and perception. No matter what science offers by way of explanation of diseases, operations and procedures, that which determines patient response is what the patient attributes to their experiences. Every individual has their own unique set of attitudes and values and these can have a profound effect on the illness experience and how patients respond. It is for that reason that person-centred care focuses so strongly upon the patient narrative (how patients relate their story of illness) and a search for answers that resonate as valuable to the patient. If we don't understand the patient's perceptions of events, then we miss the essential starting point for forthcoming care.

The second thing you might have observed is that in person-centred care the relationship between the patient and the nurse is itself therapeutic (Doherty and Thompson, 2014). The patient experiences care through the way that the nurse speaks and behaves. Conversation is no longer simply polite; it becomes itself a vehicle for improving the lot of the patient. If you work in mental health nursing, this may already be familiar. If the nursing process explains the sequence of professional work to be done, then person-centred care majors on the medium through which this is done and it is the relationship that you build (Van Belle et al., 2019). Whether treatment works, whether recovery and rehabilitation seem a success, relies in large part on the relationship that you build together.

What is less apparent in any algorithm diagram is that whether we talk about the nursing process or person-centred care, practical caring cannot be entirely described by boxes or stages. The nurse constantly checks how the patient experiences care, problems or successes with treatment. In reality, care often goes back and forth between stages of care, although first principles remain. We try to establish a relationship before we collaborate on care; it is wise to assess and plan before you act.

It can seem rather daunting – to realise that everything you say or do can mean so much! But it remains true that patients respond to and remember nurses by the manner in which they communicated, and the way that they focused upon felt needs when they were vulnerable (Saletnik, 2019; Yehudia, 2020). Think for a moment about cancer. What do you think that the patient remembers most about the nurse's care? Was it the skilful way that cytotoxic drugs were administered, a wound dressed, or do you think it was the way that the nurse allayed anxiety? Person-centred care argues that we know patients and they know us through the medium of the relationship: the way in which we manage change, threat, anxiety and hope with them. Whilst you might think this is instinctive, in person-centred care you are encouraged to explore whether it can be strategic as well.

Anticipating

We move now to each of the stages of the person-centred care process in turn, relating the same to the nursing process where appropriate and highlighting what is entailed. In Part 2 of this book case studies will illustrate this staged work in rather more detail.

Before we meet patients, we need to anticipate the commonly occurring concerns, perceptions and needs they are likely to have when they come into our care (Price, 2017). This is important because:

- there won't necessarily be time to ask them every question that might be useful at the first meeting;
- we need to build rapport with the patient, assuring them that we are already familiar with the more common concerns that often arise;
- we hope to quickly assure the patient that frequently met major problems are centre-stage in our service to them.

If you review research evidence, past patient audit and feedback on experiences of illness, treatment and care, you can then include questions at the opening interview that will strike the patient as very relevant. In short, you will seem alert to patient needs and exactly at the time when the relationship starts as one between strangers (Price, 2017). One of the important ingredients for successful person-centred care is an adequate repository of past patient experience information, whether that comes from research, audit or case study. Information of other kinds (for example, research evidence about the efficacy of different treatments) will mean little if we do not understand how patients experience and cope with illness.

Activity 2.2   Reflection

- Which evidence-searching and audit review skills do you think you will need to exercise in order to anticipate commonly recurring patient concerns and needs?
- Why do you think searches need to focus upon the patient experiences where you work?
- What do you think are the implications for clinical expertise and specialisation?

An outline answer is given at the end of this chapter.

Relating

Once we meet the patient, the business of relating begins. You have considerable lifetime experience of this – the opening of a relationship of one kind or another. Here, though, the relationship will be a professional one, something centred on countering illness or injury and which promotes health and a sense of wellbeing (Scheffelaar et al., 2019). For that reason, the relationship necessarily begins with a series of enquiries – questions about what has been happening to the patient and how this has seemed to them. Some patients may already have a medical diagnosis at this stage, but for many others there might exist a period of ambiguity, when signs and symptoms have to be made sense of (e.g. Graner et al., 2016). So our enquiries with the patient have to:

- be purposeful;
- seem respectful (a managed level of intrusion);
- focus adequately on the patient's experiences and feelings (we become a professional friend);
- enable the patient to express themselves in their own way (we must resist the temptation to box these into our own preconceptions of what is most important).

We can call this process discovering the patient narrative (Launer, 2018). Instead of focusing purely on a series of standard check questions (allergies, past admission to hospital, frequency and extent of signs or symptoms), we invite the patient to detail their experiences. Look at this short passage taken from a patient who was recounting his early experience of Covid-19 infection. Notice the emphasis on gradually evolving perceptions of what was wrong and what that meant. It is this sort of insight, into the way the patient tells their story, that improves our understanding of their needs and what they can later bring to care negotiations:

> *I started with a dry cough and you know it wasn't like a cold then. When I get a cold my sinuses fill up and my wife despairs. She hates men with colds and how miserable they become. Anyway, this was a dry cough and it was only that at first. Then I got the headaches and wow they were worse than migraines I have had in the past. My temperature must have rocketed because my shirt was soaking with sweat. It was horrible. (Dean)*

Illness for Dean was an experience of increasing concern. This illness wasn't the same as others. But it was serious – notice the comment about the headaches and sweating. Had we simply asked the patient to list their signs and symptoms, we would have missed a great deal. We need to understand how the patient feels in order to respond empathetically. I said to Dean:

> *So that seemed really threatening? [asking for clarification] How did you deal with that? [Tell me more, about coping]*

I used open questions (those that didn't easily permit a yes or no answer) to encourage Dean to portray his illness and what he did in response. The way in which Dean defines the problem or the need is an important point from which care is then negotiated.

Rapport building is not a formula. It is not a protocol to be followed, or an assessment instrument to be used. It is rather something that happens incrementally through the way questions are asked, and the way in which reflections and responses are then shared (Price, 2017). How you react to what the patient says can either encourage the patient to explain more or fall silent. The important message to convey through the conversations is that you (the patient) are very important. What you experienced is as important to me as any tests that we run. We have to listen hard and ask supplementary questions about how the patient proceeded; how they like to tackle challenges such as illness. For example, 'You said you self-medicated then. What did you take and how did you think that would help?'

From the way in which the patient recounts their experiences and feelings, you begin to sense their level of confidence, and the way in which they currently think of themselves as a patient (Page and Stritzke, 2015). Because the patient is on a journey (through illness or injury), you need to sense how far they think they have travelled and how well they are travelling. Here are some possible self-perceptions that the patient may have as you begin to relate to them:

- I'm ill but I'm coping. I just need a little help from you.
- I'm lost; I don't understand what is happening to me!
- I can't cope – this is devastating!
- This is what is wrong and this is what I am going to do about it.

When you look at a list like this it should be apparent that two important dimensions exist at this stage. The first relates to the sense of control that the patient does or doesn't have (e.g. Pauling et al., 2018). At one extreme is victimhood: the patient feels lost, powerless, confused. At the other extreme is a sense of understanding and control. In the final bullet example, the patient identifies a problem and sees themselves as a problem solver. They believe that they have the ability to address the problem before them. The second important dimension relates to certainty or otherwise about the nature of the problem, and the challenge before them (e.g. Etkind et al., 2016). The penultimate bullet point example above was voiced by a patient who was convinced that she had cancer when in fact she didn't. The perception is important because this later shapes what the nurse says to the patient; where the support might lie. Assessing

Activity 2.3 Reflection

Think back now to a patient that you have cared for and remember whether you identified their narrative.

- In retrospect, did the identification of that seem important?
- If you did identify their narrative, did you then notice anything about (a) how confident they seemed and (b) whether they were clear and accurate about what was happening to them?

As this is based on your own reflection, no outline answer is given at the end of this chapter.

the patient's confidence level and their understanding of their current circumstances begins to suggest how far they can partner us in care planning and delivery. A patient, for example, who feels emotionally paralysed by their circumstances cannot partner in care as quickly as someone who feels that they have some personal coping available. The more confident patient may seem an excellent partner in care, but challenges may still remain if they misunderstand something about their illness and treatment.

Negotiating

As in nursing process terms you move from assessment to care planning, so in person-centred terms you move from relating to negotiating. Both should produce a plan of care, based on patient consent at minimum (nurse-delivered care) and patient collaboration in ideal circumstances (jointly enacted care). In practice you will continue to enhance relationship building throughout the span of care, but for practical purposes here we will describe person-centred care in stages.

The term 'negotiate' seems to suggest that most things are open to mutual determination, affording the patient a considerable degree of power. In practice, though, this is very hard to achieve (Griscti et al., 2016). What the patient thinks desirable might not be realisable. What the patient thinks best suits his or her lifestyle might carry significant risks as identified by research evidence. Negotiation then starts with the nurse explanation of issues, risks and problems. Whilst some patients come to care vastly experienced (in chronic illness, for example), many more may come to care disadvantaged by what they do not yet understand, and sometimes by beliefs that have little foundation in science. Gently, respectfully, the nurse has to acquaint the patient with issues, risks and problems that are important to the patient's circumstances. In psychological terms we call this modelling (Albert, 2015). A problem is not something that exists separate from the patient; it takes shape from the ways in which a diagnosis and necessary treatment interact with the patient's personal circumstances. Imagine then a child that has been diagnosed with grand mal epilepsy. The problem is not simply one associated with the frequency, pattern of location of seizures and effectiveness of medication (a medical problem); it is one associated too with perceptions of fits, injury and perhaps incontinence for a child that has them in public places (a personal problem). The nurse negotiates with the patient a better understanding of the personal and the medical problem and how that might sensitively be addressed.

It is this focus on the personal problem that commends the nurse's work as person-centred, caring and imaginative. Countering that problem, however, the issue or risk has to be approached through what the patient currently understands; what they may hope for. Some things may seem more possible than others and at the outset of care negotiation it may be necessary for the nurse to acknowledge limits of service; the limit of science today; the matters as yet unresolved about a particular illness or management options (Naldemirci et al., 2020). In some instances, the patient may identify unrealistic goals. The nurse has to honestly relate what experience has so far taught us. Alternatively, a patient might lack optimism and the nurse might suggest that something more might be achievable. It is in such negotiations that the nurse tries to be wise, helping the patient to start formulating desirable and realistic goals.

Activity 2.4   Speculating

What do you think might happen as you start to uncover issues and the nature of the personal problem that the patient faces? If you have experience of dealing with difficulties in association with care negotiations, briefly jot those down.

An outline answer is given at the end of this chapter.

Whilst most textbooks on person-centred care emphasise joint planning and the identification of goals, it is necessary to clarify too the contributions to be made in pursuit of those (Price, 2017). In many healthcare circumstances there will not be one absolute and unchanging goal at the start of care, something relentlessly worked towards. Instead, there will be a series of goals that are reviewed and adjusted as care progresses. For example, a patient suffering from cancer might start with goals of appraising the illness threat (keeping it in proportion and reviewing how best to cope), but this may quickly shift to managing the side effects of treatment in a dignified way. Goals shift as care progresses. What then also shifts is how much the patient feels able to contribute to the care work and what is then required from the nurse (Elwyn et al., 2016). Classically, early acute illness care is often nurse led. The nurse does much of the care. Later, in recovery and rehabilitation, the patient is asked to contribute more care work of their own. They may manage a stoma, clean their catheter, take control of their insulin therapy. Much of the innovative person-centred care writing then centres on the later-stage relationship, where we know the patient better (e.g. Hoedemakers et al., 2019).

Whilst in some instances (for example, a patient in intensive care) there is very limited scope for the patient to contribute a great deal of care, the search for collaborative activity remains important for three reasons:

- it justifies the enquiry into the patient's narrative. Such intrusion comes with a commitment to work closely with the patient on problems afterwards;
- the success of care is rarely dependent upon just what nurses do – it is more often about how patients respond as well;
- the degree of care success may rely in part upon changing roles; what the patient feels able to contribute to. The care plan is not a catalogue of consumer demands. If it were, then the goals would need to be rather less ambitious, as healthcare resources are necessarily limited.

Activity 2.5   Critical thinking

Care plans classically describe a problem, need or nursing diagnosis, identify one or more attendant goals, outline activity designed to achieve the goal, and include relevant review dates so that care seems disciplined (Gulanick and Myers, 2017).

What do you think might be rather different then about a person-centred plan of care? Jot your ideas down before reading on.

As this activity is based on your own reflection, there is no outline answer at the end of this chapter.

I wonder how you responded to Activity 2.5? Some of the nurses I have worked with have emphasised that the care plan in person-centred care is remarkably similar to that which is written in the nursing care process. Both need to be clear as regards goals and actions and both need planned timescales for work. The nursing care goals and activity often signal a sequence of work: what will be done first, second and third. Some elements of care might proceed in parallel and sometimes there may be a need to include review points, especially if screening and tests have yet to confirm a diagnosis and suggest possible treatment options. Thus far the person-centred care plan and that routinely written in the nursing process have many similarities.

There are, however, differences too, and these centre on the fact that personal problems (how the patient experiences illness or treatment) need to feature just as much as medical problems (those that centre more abstractly on the disease process, for instance). So in person-centred care the problem will be framed in the context of the patient's circumstances as well as attend to clinical considerations. For example, a problem linked to newly diagnosed Type 2 diabetes mellitus would not simply state the imbalance of food intake to insulin supply and energy needs; it would relate it in terms of the patient's personal lifestyle.

I need to find ways of managing my insulin therapy that work with my job shifts and exercise schedule.

In this example the problem and the goal (to achieve a balance) quickly come together and are expressed as a need. This is because the patient owns the challenge of diabetes in their own terms. Their body might need to balance insulin and food intake, sustaining energy requirements of the body (a medical problem), but the patient needs to manage all of that whilst sustaining a viable lifestyle (a personal problem). Writing problems and goals in firmly personal-circumstance terms emphasises to the patient that this is their plan of care too (Christie et al., 2020). It reinforces the importance of their control when responding to illness or injury. Typically, then, in person-centred care the patient retains the care plan and may add notes or concerns that they later wish to consult the nurse upon. The care plan is not something that is guarded by the nurse, or kept separate from the patient. The care plan has scope for patient or lay carer comment, a place where notes can be added as care progresses. Whilst the nurse may have drafted the plan of care with the patient's consent, it doesn't remain a nurse-only document for update.

This approach is significantly different from environments where all care and treatment records are stored within a ward office or a departmental record station. Care planning in this way becomes truly coherent when not only nurses but also doctors and other therapists make contributions to the plan. That has significant implications as regards diagnosis and decisions about when and how patients are appraised of what tests and investigations reveal. You may have already reflected that some care work, screening, testing and differential diagnosis review is necessarily carried out away from the patient. To subject them to all the possible diagnoses during a process of elimination could cause significant distress. For that reason, then, compromises are usually found with medical contributions to the care plan increasing only when a diagnosis has been arrived at and treatment options discussed with the patient.

Not every patient may wish to engage this deeply with the care planning process, at least at the point where a plan is first recorded. This might seem a person-centred care failure to you, but remember what was argued in Chapter 1. Patients retain significant control over the care process and that includes the right to say that they wish the nurse to direct more of their care. It is possible, therefore, that the nursing care plan becomes an evolving document, one where patient contribution increases over time. What the nurse has first written and had checked by the patient may incrementally become something that the patient later adds notes to. What remains important, however, is that the patient feels regularly and fully consulted upon as care is planned and then delivered.

Collaborating

Despite what is taught within nursing courses on campus about care philosophy, many nurses' experience of care-giving is relatively task-orientated (Havaei et al., 2019). This is because nursing shifts are divided up into a series of set-time activities that have to be completed diligently and sometimes in a particular sequence. The nursing day, for instance, is punctuated by meal times, by medicine rounds, by observations (physiological and psychological), by dressings and other treatments and by consultation between ourselves, patients and medical colleagues. Whilst such arrangements enable the working day to seem predictable and efficient, they rob the nurse of an equally important focus upon the care relationship, which shifts somewhat day to day dependent on what is happening to the patient and how they are coping. We can too easily lose focus upon the patient and attend instead to the healthcare system.

In person-centred care this tendency to slip towards the system-operative mindset is partially offset by thinking quite specifically about the roles we might adopt with different patients as their illness or disability is managed (e.g. Brown et al., 2016). In Chapter 1

I alluded to a relative balance of care: that which the patient contributes and that which the nurse provides. Now, though, we need to consider how the nurse's contribution might be arranged. What is it that we actually do and how is that demonstrated in the way that we talk to and listen to patients? Person-centred care nurses adopt roles and subset ways of thinking and working as the routine scheduled events of the nursing day proceed. Rest assured, drugs are still administered, dressings completed, patients assisted to eat a meal, physiological and psychological observations made and individual/family/group therapy carried out, but the manner in which the nurse collaborates with the patient changes dependent upon the role adopted.

Activity 2.6   Speculating

Imagine now a patient with a problem that is fairly commonly encountered in your current field of work or clinical placement. Now jot down the roles that you think you already play in supporting them. Add to that list any additional roles that you believe might improve their care if resources seemed sufficient and you were confident that you had the requisite skills.

An outline answer is given at the end of this chapter.

Sometimes nurses think of roles as something rather grand and associated with additional training and qualification. Many roles, however, are rather more modest and you might already think of them as skills that you have been taught on your course of studies. Listening, for instance, is certainly a skill – we have to actively hear what the patient says and encourage them to share their thoughts fully – but being a listener is also a role (Weiner and Schwartz, 2016). During the collaborative stage of person-centred care we adopt roles that advanced the care goals we have negotiated. So imagine that you are currently supporting a very anxious patient. Being the listener right now is extremely important as the patient explores the extent and nature of their anxieties. You will endeavour first to help the patient map their anxieties and then to judge whether all of those are entirely realistic. Some anxieties can be quickly allayed; others demand much more attention and support.

What is unique to person-centred care is the extent to which we adopt roles that seem to quickly and sensitively address patient felt needs. The patient senses how intuitive we seem, adopting roles that seem to perfectly match their requirements. A patient might say, 'I don't know how you read me so fast. You always seem to appreciate what it feels like to be dealing with all this'. The roles that we adopt then are relatively dynamic; they don't remain rigid for all time and usually they complement the role of the patient. If we teach, then the patient learns, and we had better make sure that we understand what learning feels like!

At other times our adopted roles are chosen in response to the medical problem – that which the patient has to confront. So, for example, the youngster who has developed grand mal epilepsy will need some teaching to master his medication, and to understand what to do if he experiences warning that a fit is about to develop. He will need to learn about whether the fits seem associated with other things, for instance his level of tiredness. Teaching is a major skill in nursing because it helps to shift power back to the patient, to give them what Orem described as increased 'self-care agency' (in Sassen, 2017). Some of the roles adopted by nurses then deal with what is irrefutable – an illness that demands some sort of adjustment in the patient's lifestyle.

Activity 2.7   Reflection

Look back now to the possible nurse roles that were summarised in Table 1.3 of Chapter 1 (p17). Which of these roles seems especially relevant to the patient that you thought about again in Activity 2.6? Are there roles there that you would like to know more about and which might form a focus for your portfolio reading?

As this activity is based on your own reflection, no outline answer is given at the end of this chapter.

Before leaving role-based activity, it seems important to acknowledge the potential for conflict in care – situations where the role adopted by the nurse seems less welcomed by the patient. Care does not always run smoothly and ethical issues can arise, for instance, where stakeholders contest decisions (Teeri et al., 2016). Some patients may staunchly resist an invitation from the nurse to partner in care. Person-centred care is a psychological form of work. It includes exploring the patient's experiences, perceptions, needs, values and attitudes. People develop values and attitudes over time and they are strongly linked to a personal sense of identity (Galliher et al., 2017). Where illness or treatment challenge the patient to question their current values and attitudes, conflict may arise for the patient (e.g. Carter et al., 2018). It takes time for patients to come to terms with their new health circumstances. A patient who has been told that they are dying, for instance, may for a considerable period of time refuse to believe that it is true. Person-centred care cannot compel patients to believe particular things; it cannot coerce them to behave in health-beneficial ways. The ethical stance adopted is one of wise counselling, where the nurse advises the patient (or their guardians) of the merits and the risks or limits of different courses of action.

Were the nurse to avoid such complex and taxing situations, to simply complete tasks with the patient, to deliver the required information about an illness or treatment, nursing work might seem much less stressful. We might simply observe that we have explained the necessary evidence, or delivered the standardised care mandated. But person-centred care tries to work more intimately with patient felt needs and beliefs.

It does so because we believe that substantial and sustainable change may become possible that way. That means that in delivering care this way it will be important to consult regularly with colleagues on whether care is working well. Person-centred care nurses experience a range of doubts about the collaborative care that they deliver. As well as consulting the patient on what seems welcome, they need the support of colleagues where it seems necessary to persevere with care work that seems imperative to the medical problem.

Care work requires effort on the part of both the nurse and the patient and it is by no means certain that this will always run well. Collaborating with patients then requires frequent monitoring to judge how well care is proceeding. In the nursing process that monitoring classically focuses on whether the patient's condition is improving and whether nurse contributions seem effective. In person-centred care, however, there is an additional emphasis upon patient morale and confidence (Price, 2017). If within person-centred nursing the patient has greater control of care, then they also feel the weight of maintaining progress. Patients who are ill may already be prone to self-doubt about their coping. The status quo within their lives has been disrupted. The person-centred care nurse remains alert to how the patient continues to narrate their experience of illness, treatment and any recovery or rehabilitation work that they contribute.

Pause to think about why patient morale and motivation seems this important in person-centred care. Why do you think that we are quite so concerned about how the patient narrates their continuing journey? The answer rests largely within the life-changing goals that attend person-centred care. Nurses not only wish to deliver care that seems more humane and respectful; they also wish to enrich the life that the patient then leads. Many patients will have to live with a chronic illness. They may need to continue with treatment for the rest of their lives. If they are to sustain that lifelong effort, then, it is important in early care that the nurse successfully identifies that which could undermine patient confidence. Investments in understanding the patient and their motivation now may well pay long-term dividends if the patient then goes on to successfully manage their illness. Understanding the patient well, how hope could falter, what undermines their resolve, may play a vital role in reducing the need for subsequent hospital admissions and perhaps later corrective treatment.

Activity 2.8   Reflection

Identify now, within your own field of practice, healthcare conditions where there are common problems in sustaining long-term independence. Now reflect on why the person-centred care emphasis on patient psychology and monitoring of morale and motivation seems especially valuable there.

I offer brief reflections of my own at the end of this chapter.

Evaluating

We come at last to evaluating care. In the person-centred context, this involves both the patient and the nurse reviewing not only what was achieved, but also what was learned along the way (Newton et al., 2019). At its best, person-centred care enables people to determine what they learned from the roles they fulfilled and the goals and care activities that they conferred upon. There is an emphasis on what I did, what we did and what we changed. There is also an emphasis upon where we have arrived now. This last point is especially important because whilst the evaluation work is often completed just prior to patient discharge from hospital, in reality, evaluation often focuses upon work that remains in progress. The patient continues to learn to self-care. He or she may have to work with new healthcare professionals and avail themselves of different services. The nurse at this stage might conclude that care relationship, but there will be others to follow and case experience becomes the anticipation stage of future person-centred care. Every evaluation has the potential to teach the nurse something about how they relate to patients.

In person-centred care, evaluation takes account of the opening patient narrative, about their illness and circumstances. What has the shared care done to that narrative? Is the patient less anxious and more confident that they have the means to cope successfully? Has a new narrative replaced the old one, hopefully one that accentuates trust in the nurse and what they can do to help? The narrative may yet be in transition, the patient identifying further work to do, in which case the nurse acts as a consultant, advising the patient where further guidance might be sought. At the end of this stage in care, completely new goals might emerge. When I worked at the Royal Marsden Hospital patients dealing with cancer frequently reported new objectives, and better ways to live once they had achieved remission from their illness. They were entirely aware that remission did not necessarily mean a cure. For that reason, the threat of cancer prompted a new way to value daily activities, to accentuate that which seemed more important to them and their families.

One of the things I learned about person-centred care was that evaluation often highlights changing perceptions of one another – the nurse and the patient. Confronted with the major threat of illness and perhaps an unclear prognosis, patients find it much harder to cope in a familiar way. Illness can be terrifying and it is in such stressful circumstances patients and nurses negotiate care. Both patients and nurses learn about themselves and in doing so they may re-evaluate how they have viewed each other. Here is a paraphrase of what one woman said to me after undergoing radical surgery for cancer of her mouth.

> *You clearly wanted me to learn new ways to think of myself even though I felt like curling up in a ball. When you started that way, it didn't seem very kind. Then I started to ask what I wanted for myself after the surgery was done. I started to wonder how best to respond to others and the way they react to me. Then you became something else, more of a counsellor. You seemed gentler.*

The evaluation is quite frank and in truth I could not be sure that my opening teaching stance was a wise one. But the point had been that this woman's opening narrative had emphasised her rational problem-solving approach to life. She thought of herself as someone who coped by adapting. After diagnosis and as treatment progressed, she had significant doubts about that ability. I hoped to sustain that coping approach until she could become inquisitive and self-starting again. Later this woman mentored others who had undergone radical maxofacial surgery associated with cancer. On this occasion the nursing support had worked, although it was not vouchsafed always to do so. The chances of its success were predicated upon what was already known from her opening narrative about herself.

Chapter summary

In this chapter we have highlighted aspects of person-centred care in process – that which relates closely to the care relationship. We have set this out as a series of stages. In many ways, the process replicates the disciplined and methodical nature of the nursing process, but it acknowledges too a certain untidiness as the nurse tries to understand the patient's narrative and then to use that to negotiate care that seems meaningful and acceptable to the patient. There will always be degrees of person-centred care. Patients may be more or less ready to partner the nurse in problem analysis and care planning. Where, however, patients do feel able to share a person-centred care relationship, there is considerable scope for each to learn from the other. We move on now to examine some case studies of person-centred care in process.

Activities: Brief outline answers

Activity 2.2 Reflection (p28)

A full discussion of evidence reviewing can be found in the companion volume by Price (2021), *Critical Thinking and Writing in Nursing*. In summary, though, you will need to employ relevant search terms, typically including the illness or problem (e.g. 'diabetes mellitus Type 2') and the focus on patient experience or need (e.g. 'patient coping' or 'patient needs'). Whilst other research evidence on treating this condition is important, in person-centred care you need to cover patient experiences. After that you will need a quizzical attitude to the qualitative data and report presented. This sort of research illustrates needs and problems; it doesn't prescribe solutions. Your local patients may have other additional or alternative concerns that you know about from past experience. The focus upon patient experience is important because we want to signal our interest in patient felt needs. What all of this signifies for local practice is that nurses need to stay abreast of field-specific research and audit evidence – that which relates to their particular patients.

Activity 2.4 Speculating (p32)

It is sometimes surprising to discover just how different patient expectations of nurses, and nursing care, are to our own. However much we wish to offer a partnership in care to patients, it sometimes transpires that this invitation is not accepted. Whatever the nursing philosophy is, patients start with their own agendas, and in some instances that includes a more distant working relationship with the nurse. Another possible surprise is that patient expectations are suddenly revealed; those that seem overwhelming. Some patients are angry and disgruntled about healthcare, perhaps because of past experiences. Person-centred care feels more intimate, and our ability to deliver that care depends on what the patient feels happy to negotiate. I recommend that you consult colleagues if you discover that the patient rejects your invitation to partner in care or else demands unrealistic provision. It is better to assess a workable relationship at the start than to promise what you cannot deliver.

A relatively frequent discovery is that patients understand the origins of problems differently to you – this may be informed by folk beliefs about disease. You quickly become aware that research evidence is different to what the patient believes happens. This will pose a challenge as you consider how to gently counter misunderstandings and bring valuable information to their attention. Clearly, an abrupt 'let me stop you there, that's an old wives' tale' is unlikely to help build rapport. You will need to gently explore the origins of the patient's ideas before you acquaint them with alternative research accounts of how an illness arises or develops.

Activity 2.6 Speculating (p35)

Some years ago I worked regularly with patients who had been burned. The medical problem was one of stabilising their fluid balance, managing pain and avoiding infection within their wounds. It was very physiological. But the personal problem was very much about altered body image, an overwhelming psychological shock as the patient confronted their new appearance or function. So, my opening role with the patient was one of psychological support, helping them to map the change and to grieve for their changed circumstances. After that my role shifted and I taught them how to evaluate their self-worth differently, valuing psychological strengths that they could deploy with others in explaining their new appearance.

Activity 2.8 Reflection (p37)

Person-centred care majors on the psychological and acts as a counterbalancing weight to physical care, which can come to dominate many fields of practice. Often, modern medicine cannot offer a cure to patients, but it can offer tools to mitigate the effects of an illness or injury (e.g. medications). Whether the patient fully avails themselves of these resources depends upon their health beliefs – that which motivate the patient. Person-centred care works quickly and intimately with beliefs and values, facilitating lifestyle change that may well increase the patient's independence long term and help save the health service significant money otherwise spent on corrective measures. Put rather simply, the person-centred care emphasis on perceptions, narratives and collaboration becomes a good long-term investment for patients and service alike.

Further reading

McCormack, B, Van Dulman, S, Eide, H et al. (2017) *Person-Centred Healthcare Research.* Chichester: John Wiley and Sons.

Brendan McCormack and colleagues have written extensively on the philosophy of person-centred care. You will gain insights into why nurses are so interested in patient experiences and narratives and why the development of new nursing skills is important for the person-centred care nurse.

Muller, R (2018) *Trauma and the Struggle to Open Up: From Avoidance to Recovery and Growth.* New York: W.B. Norton and Company.

Person-centred care nurses are not psychotherapists. There are always patients that need a prompt referral to specialist psychological help. But nurses who practise person-centred care routinely encounter patients who are struggling with their illness or injury, making sense of their circumstances. So a book like this is an excellent read if only to reassure yourself that sometimes when a patient doesn't partner you in care, it is because they are simply not ready to.

Useful websites

Understanding narratives in health care. OpenLearn, The Open University.

This free-to-download resource produced by the Open University explores the different meanings of narrative and how they shape not only how patients behave but healthcare staff as well. I would suggest that if person-centred nursing care starts anywhere, it is with an ability to listen to patients and a good understanding of their narratives, so this is well worth accessing. Visit www.open.edu, select OpenLearn and then search 'Understanding narratives in health care'.

Richards, T (2014) Listen to patients: how Radboud UMC changed quality and care. *British Medical Journal*, doi: 10.1136/bmj.g5765

This reference will link you directly to a *British Medical Journal* podcast on person-centred care in the Netherlands, describing the change in service mindset that helped to engage patients as partners in nursing care but also a wider service beyond. Doctors too are interested in person-centred care and understand the alienating effects of hospital on patients, especially upon first admission. The resource comes from 2014 but I think that the upbeat analysis remains as pertinent today as then.

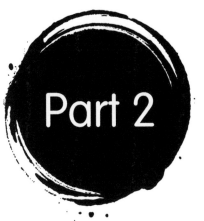

Part 2   How to deliver person-centred care

Part 2 of this textbook presents four case studies, each of which highlights aspects of person-centred nursing care over the course of a patient's healthcare journey. The case studies are based on real-life patient care episodes and expressed needs, although particular aspects of care have been picked out to help you to relate the theory of person-centred care to practice. The case studies serve a heuristic purpose, to help you tease out person-centred nursing care in action. Replacement names have been used in each of the case studies to protect the privacy of patients, relatives and healthcare staff concerned.

The case studies are presented from four different fields of nursing practice, namely: adult, children, learning disabilities and mental health. It will quickly become apparent, however, that patients' needs are not so readily partitioned by such divisions; a patient may have both physical and mental healthcare needs, for instance.

It would be erroneous to pretend that any case study personifies perfect person-centred care. Each offers elements of good practice. What represents the very best person-centred care is determined by patients, relatives and nurses finding the best-fit ways forward. Throughout the case study chapters I pose reflective practice activities for you to complete and these include reflection about what you have witnessed, done or previously speculated about. Each of the case studies include insights into person-centred care and best practice tips in conclusion.

In Chapter 3 we meet Abraham, a 65-year-old man suffering from the effects of Covid-19 infection and transiting through intensive care and on into recovery. The case study has been selected because in such acute-care settings it is especially difficult to demonstrate person-centred care. Here you have a chance to reflect on the care environment as well as to examine how the stages in a care relationship develop. The account centres on care before and after mechanical ventilation as these are places where perceptions, expressed needs and concerns can help shape care delivery.

In Chapter 4 we meet John, in his 60s, who has a learning disability and who is confronted with the need to undergo elective surgery because of bowel cancer.

John provides an opportunity for you to explore care liaison between nurses and friends and to examine how a care environment might be made more person-friendly.

In Chapter 5 we turn to the field of children's nursing and a 14-year-old boy called Tom. Tom has developed diabetes mellitus and will have to manage a chronic illness for the rest of his life. Diabetes is a significant medical challenge, one that poses very personal problems for a young person as they contemplate how best to live well. This case study explains how teaching and learning might be conceived as part of person-centred care.

In the last case study (Chapter 6), attention shifts to Susan, a patient dealing with depression, and focuses in particular on the challenge of motivating the patient to sustain effective self-care. Person-centred care is especially valuable in mental health nursing where communication is itself conceived as therapeutic.

Each of the case studies have been presented using the staged relationship headings of person-centred care that you met in Part 1 of the book (anticipating, relating, negotiating, collaborating and evaluating). The emphasis placed on each stage will depend upon insights available, but each case study will provide an overview of person-centred care as a process. To assist you I match the stage section headings of the person-centred care relationship to those of the nursing process (in brackets). Please remember, though, that care tends to shift back and forth. No care relationship is rigidly linear and earlier stages of care work are sometimes revisited to revise a plan of care.

Part 2 of the book is concluded with a final chapter taking stock and looking forward to person-centred care in the future.

Chapter 3

Case study one

Helping Abraham survive Covid-19

NMC Future Nurse Standards of Proficiency for Registered Nurses

This chapter will address the following platforms and proficiencies:

Platform 1: Being an accountable professional

At the point of registration the registered nurse will be able to:

1.8   demonstrate the knowledge, skills and ability to think critically when applying evidence and drawing on experience to make evidence-informed decisions in all situations.

Platform 2: Promoting health and preventing ill health

At the point of registration, the registered nurse will be able to:

2.10   provide information in accessible ways to help people understand and make decisions about their health, life choices, illness and care.

Platform 3: Assessing needs and planning care

At the point of registration, the registered nurse will be able to:

3.5   demonstrate the ability to accurately process all information gathered during the assessment process to identify needs for individualised nursing care and develop person-centred evidence-based plans for nursing interventions with agreed goals.

> ## Chapter aims
>
> After reading this chapter you will be able to:
>
> - review the ways in which evidence, standardised care provision and person-centred care might combine when delivering care to a patient;
> - discuss the modifications to person-centred care that might be necessary when a patient is acutely ill and cannot readily negotiate care;
> - explore the person-centred care stages and how care work may then vary in each, dependent on the patient's ability to partner the nurse in care.

Introduction

It is hard to imagine a situation less conducive to person-centred care than the support of a patient experiencing the severe respiratory effects of Covid-19 infection. The illness seems daunting as patients may become seriously ill very quickly, limiting time to express individual needs before some are then supported on a ventilator. Abraham, the 65-year-old gentleman who features in this case study, experienced a 24-hour period of fever, dry cough and fatigue, before dyspnoea rapidly took over and he was admitted to the district hospital. Over two days his respiratory condition deteriorated and he was then intubated and put on a mechanical ventilator. Abraham spent a total of six days on the ventilator before he was returned to an oxygen regime using nasal cannula. Ten days post-weaning from the ventilator, Abraham left the district hospital, at which point the case study period concludes. Abraham was cared for by a series of nurses, each of whom offers part of the illustration of person-centred care in action. For some of the time (whilst mechanically ventilated) Abraham remained oblivious to the care that was provided. On the admissions ward he was severely ill and found it difficult to relate to Personal Protection Equipment (PPE)-clad nurses in the ways that we might ideally hope. In some regards, the personal relationship then only really blossomed as he recovered from his time on the Intensive Care Unit. Much of the frontloaded care was delivered in a way that met anticipated needs but was not open to much negotiation. At the start of Abraham's care, evidence-based care and a standard care package (that was deemed to reduce risk of death) was in the ascendency. Only later could the person-centred care approach move convincingly to centre-stage.

This chapter will explore the context of the case study (what you need to appreciate) and the story of the patient, and then lead you through each of the person-centred care stages. In this and indeed all of the case study chapters, we will then pick out the key insights it offers on what seems important about person-centred care.

Covid-19 viral pandemic

Whilst the date of the first Covid-19 outbreak cases is debated, by the beginning of 2020 the World Health Organization (WHO) declared that a global pandemic was underway (Brown and Ladwig, 2020). Covid-19 is believed to have originated in bats and successfully transferred to human beings. The viral infection is spread via droplet/aerosol means and, like other viruses of the coronavirus group, is prone to mutate in ways that make it increasingly transmissible (Gandhi et al., 2020). The initial reports of healthcare problems came from Wuhan in China and the profile of illness consisted of a high fever, fatigue, dry cough, increasing dyspnoea, chills and, in some cases, problems affecting the patient's sense of smell and gastrointestinal system (diarrhoea) (Keller et al., 2020). Younger people contracting Covid-19 in particular might remain asymptomatic, or else experience minor flu-like symptoms, but in older adults, the infection might rapidly produce more severe respiratory difficulties and pneumonia. Patients who were obese, male, from minority-ethnic communities and suffering from a compromised immune system were especially at risk, and amongst those a relatively small percentage of infections (circa 5%) led to Acute Respiratory Distress Syndrome (ARDS), septicaemia, multiple organ failure and death (Zhou et al., 2020). Despite the low percentage of patients advancing to severe illness, the preponderance of an ageing population in the UK and elsewhere meant that in the spring of 2020 healthcare services were severely tested. Patients were at first treated with oxygen and artificial ventilation and those surviving then faced extended periods of rehabilitation as fatigue and dyspnoea slowly abated over a period of weeks or months. During the course of 2020 healthcare science announced ways in which treatments for other conditions might be repurposed to fight Covid-19. Repurposed treatments included antiviral agents, corticosteroids such as dexamethasone and most recently beta interferon (Johnson, 2020; Pascarella et al., 2020; Seavone et al., 2020).

Public health measures, organised as lockdowns, were successful in countering the first wave of the pandemic, reducing the rate of viral spread. In October 2020, however, a second wave of the pandemic began, this time accelerated by more transmissible variants of the virus (Jakhmola et al., 2020). A number of promising vaccines were rapidly developed and trialled and the first of these were administered in December 2020 (Public Health England, 2020).

At the time of this case study (early in the second wave of the Covid-19 pandemic in the UK), there was a greater appreciation of the likely severe illness course of the disease, with some patients developing ARDS and septicaemia (e.g. Mahdevi, 2020). Better lung perfusion had been achieved, nursing ventilated patients predominantly in the prone position (Maedo et al., 2021). Prognosis had started to improve, but the risk of death for an older man such as Abraham remained very real. Abraham, like other patients on the unit, received daily low-level doses of dexamethasone (6 mgs/day) (Johnson, 2020), designed to stave off extreme immune response (the cytokine storm) that increases the risk of death.

Case study: Abraham

Abraham is a 65-year-old man who for the recent decades of his life has worked as a security guard. Abraham works predominantly at night, driving around sites that he has to check. In recent years his relatively sedentary lifestyle and fast-food dietary habit has meant that he has become obese. At the time that Covid-19 struck, Abraham weighed a little over 20 stones (130 kilograms). Both his body weight and working pattern have arguably contributed to the risks of illness linked to Covid-19. As a night worker, Abraham has had less chance to synthesise vitamin D, that obtained via the skin from sunlight and important to immune system health (Wilson et al., 2017). Abraham's diet does not include any dietary supplements and he drinks moderate amounts of alcohol, which is also believed to have a negative effect on an individual's immune system (Pasala et al., 2015).

Abraham's health history to date has been relatively uneventful except for childhood asthma, which limited his participation in school sports. During his youth he routinely used inhalers to counter asthma attacks, although he admits that he was not consistent in taking maintenance therapy. In the last 20 years Abraham has not used an inhaler. However, he has until retirement last year been a moderate cigarette smoker, smoking 20 cigarettes a day.

Abraham is married to Lillian, who is aged 70. Lillian worked as a postal worker but found her work increasingly difficult because of the effects of osteoarthritis in her hips and spine. They live in a modest terraced house in the east end of London and Abraham describes his day as watching television, tending an allotment and listening to his wife complain. Abraham's reaction to the pandemic has been one of alarm. He has read that his cigarette smoking and weight put him at greater risk from the virus. In consequence he has limited his social contact with others, but insisted on regularly seeing his son, who has faced mental health difficulties after being made redundant from work. When Abraham began to feel unwell, Lillian insisted that it was probably influenza, but Abraham feared the worst.

Activity 3.1   Reflection

Think now about all that you have read about Covid-19 infection. Abraham's profile is high risk, but how does this become a personal problem for Abraham as well as a medical one?

Remember, personal problems centre on personal living circumstances and perceptions of threat. It's about circumstances – how something feels and what it means for living. A medical problem centres more on statistical risk and the likely impact upon the body.

An outline answer is given at the end of this chapter.

Anticipating person-centred care

Olive is the State Registered Nurse who first met Abraham upon admission to hospital and who led his care in the two days whilst his breathing became increasingly difficult. She cared for Abraham on what had once been an orthopaedic ward, but which had rapidly filled with Covid-19-infected patients. Of a cheerful and positive disposition, Olive, a Ghanaian nurse, was exhausted by the relentless pace and volume of care requirements from the patients, but she has endeavoured to convey a real sense of concern for each of them. I asked Olive about her efforts to support Abraham. To what extent was it possible to deliver person-centred care, and if she managed that, what example could she offer of the way in which care was personalised? As was explained in Part 1 of this book, person-centred care begins with anticipation. The better nurses are able to understand the likely needs of patients, the more they can demonstrate care that seems personal and attentive. Anticipated patient experiences and needs help to focus the nurse's opening enquiries. In this instance, however, Olive was working on a ward that had previously served patients undergoing hip and knee replacements. She was not in this field of care, routinely updating on respiratory healthcare challenges. There seemed less opportunity to anticipate the personal needs of a patient like Abraham.

> *The risk is that you see patients as problems, and that would be the first mistake. People like Abraham are not another chest, not another viral risk for yourself. They are more than gasping bodies. Just as before patients were not hips, so Abraham was more than a set of damaged lungs.*

The sentiment seemed professional, but surely there were real limits to care? Olive explained that she had been delivering person-centred care with people needing artificial hip joints. So the philosophy was familiar to her. But now, in a crisis, she had to tailor what she could offer to patients. She recalled what she had learned about Maslow's hierarchy of needs whilst training as a nurse (Maslow, 1954; Smith, 2017). The most fundamental needs were physiological (the need to secure enough oxygen) and after that the need to feel safe and secure. Feelings of belonging, self-esteem and self-actualisation came later and were unlikely to be met in the crisis environment that she was caring within.

> *Those two baseline needs, they aren't open to a great deal of discussion, the patients are frightened and demand oxygen. This disease scares my patients and there is no debating the matter. But I did remember something that I learned from before. You can say things whilst doing practical care that assure patients that you think about them as a person. So with Abraham I explained how oxygen would help, how nursing him upright helped him to fill his lungs. Patients don't know about lobes of the lung, so simple explanations matter. Abraham said that he used to smoke, he was worried, so I assured him that the supply of oxygen was safe. You work with the here and the now, rather than try to debate what might happen in the days to come.*

Abraham had been anxious about being admitted to hospital. For him, healthcare staff operated in a 'viral soup'. He was extremely reluctant to be admitted to hospital, fearing that the virus would quickly overwhelm him. He was also fearful that he would never see Lillian again because the no visiting policy of the hospital in Covid times was absolute. Because Lillian struggled to mobilise and would be alone, Abraham begged to be sent home with an oxygen cylinder. I asked Olive whether she remembered that? Olive explained:

> *Abraham was frightened so I said that I wouldn't leave him and that this was the best place to be. Being in hospital was where he could have oxygen and help assessing his breathing. I didn't want to scare Abraham, not all patients are moved to ICU, but I did need to help him understand some risks. So as well as talking about his smoking, his age and being heavier I reminded him that asthma wasn't just about past damage to the lungs. If you have asthma then you potentially have a bigger reaction to allergens and that might mean that his virus-affected lungs became inflamed that much more quickly [Yao et al., 2020]. I explained that his blood results showed that he was taking some time to dampen down the inflammation in his lungs and that made his breathing worse. You can't detail a cytokine storm to someone like Abraham when they're struggling to absorb so much information, but you do need to justify being near to support facilities. Whilst oxygen at home might help with breathing, we couldn't monitor him there. Abraham's blood oxygen saturation levels were dropping quickly. I explained to him that he had a high white cell count, but that his lymphocyte level had fallen. The lymphocytes are the 'good guys' that stop your lungs becoming too inflamed. This could mean that he might need more breathing assistance very soon.*

It's worth pausing at this juncture to reflect on several points in Olive's testimony of concern for Abraham. The first point to make is that Olive is clearly thinking about Abraham's capacity to understand complex information under extreme duress. If we are stressed, our ability to reason and make decisions is likely to be impaired. Olive registers that through the expression on Abraham's face, his worries and the urgent way that he clenched her hand as he gasped out questions. In shock, patients process information much less effectively. Olive searches for more accessible ways to explain things to Abraham. But there is something even more important here and it relates to the use of evidence. I wonder if you can identify what that is?

Activity 3.2   Speculating

Jot down what you think the role of evidence is in this situation. How do you think that Olive is translating evidence so that it specifically serves Abraham's needs?

Once you have jotted some points down, read on to my observations below.

As this activity is based on your own reflection, there is no outline answer given at the end of this chapter.

Olive is using evidence from her Covid-19 briefings that the hospital provided in the summer. Preparation is important if nurses are to have the right information to share with patients. That evidence refers to risk profiles, about those patients most likely to deteriorate quickly and require additional respiratory support. Whilst the news media had already indicated the general risk profile of those likely to become more seriously ill, refinements in evidence review after the first wave helped nurses to understand risk that much more. Thevarajan et al. (2020), for example, suggested parameters for which patients can be treated and monitored at home, which need to be admitted to hospital and which need transfer to the ICU. Abraham has a risk profile associated with past auto-immune hyperactivity (asthma), but also clinically associated with rapidly dropping oxygen blood saturation levels and the apparent failure of a timely lymphocyte response to help fight the infection and dampen inflammation down within the lungs. A rising white cell count and a poor lymphocyte response might signal an increased risk of ARDS and a cytokine storm (Fathi and Rezaei, 2020). The evidence is firmly medical, clinical and scientific in nature and it needed to be conveyed to the patient in a form that caused minimal distress but that nonetheless helped him to understand the advice to stay in hospital. Olive offered a rationale for staying in hospital, which was both based on Abraham's risk profile and conveyed in a way that understood his burgeoning anxieties.

It is worth thinking about this. Sometimes person-centred care is characterised as not about the volume of care that the nurse delivers, or about the scope to change care options through negotiation. In this instance, it was about drawing on evidence and translating that for a patient so that it served their circumstances well. That Olive managed to do this whilst helping Abraham with his oxygen worries is highly professional. Nurses translate evidence. They take that which is complex and relate it in more accessible terms, meeting the needs of the patient. Whilst there is a risk of misrepresenting evidence, dumbing explanations down, in extreme circumstances such as this Olive finds a commendable compromise, that which assures Abraham why he is in the right place now. She protects Abraham without unduly alarming him about clinical possibilities.

Practice tip

Don't assume that research evidence can be related stat to patients; you will need to select the most important points and convey these with regard to the patient's emotional state.

Relating and person-centred care (assessing)

In Abraham's case study, relating as a stage happened twice. The first relating began with Olive on the admissions ward. There was then a temporary hiatus in relating whilst Abraham was cared for unconscious on a ventilator. Whilst in the ICU the nurses practised with Abraham's best interests centre-stage; there was no scope to explore his perceptions or to negotiate care in such circumstances. The more familiar form of relating and rapport building then returned as he rehabilitated post-ICU. As Chapter 1 indicated, relating involves listening, narrative analysis and rapport building. If Abraham's continuity of care is threatened as he moves through different care settings (admissions ward, ICU and then rehabilitation ward), was there a thread of relationship building that was still possible? In the admissions ward there was relatively little chance for Olive and her colleagues to develop the relationship opening with Abraham very far. This was because:

- there was an overwhelming number of very ill patients, each with their own specific demands;
- patients were highly stressed, making it harder for nurses to calmly ascertain their needs;
- nurses were exhausted, making it much harder to contemplate more than what seemed the 'essentials of care';
- Abraham's stay on the admission ward was relatively short. Like some other patients of his age and risk profile, it became necessary to move him to the ICU quite quickly.

I asked Olive whether she felt that she had a personal relationship with Abraham. Was he known to her as a person? She observed that the ethos of care remained highly personal. Assistance with oral hygiene and washing, for example, was done gently, with obvious concern for the patient's discomfort and his energy deficits, but she conceded that it was much harder to know a great deal about Abraham. Patients quickly became breathless and distressed if they were asked many questions, so it seemed entirely inappropriate to quiz patients at any great length. Questions had to be focused and it was necessary to seize on snippets of information that the patient felt able to give.

Practice tip

Much information can be gathered from patients incrementally, whilst delivering physical care. Don't assume that person-centred care always begins with a lengthy interview. Interrogating a dyspnoeic patient would not assure them of your regard for them.

Olive and I discussed the compromises that were then made. The conversation revealed a rapport-building thread that she had not considered at any great length but which I suggest deserves recognition. It was Olive's practice to learn the name of the patient's spouse or other partner, the better to signal that the patient was important as a person beyond the confines of the hospital. Learning very briefly about the partner and how the patient felt about that person signalled a normality of concern about what it meant to be human that was important in exceptional circumstances. Abraham, like others, feared dying in hospital and he feared too for what that would mean for Lillian. He couldn't receive visits but he could make requests that his wife was kept well informed about what was happening to him. Abraham wished to convey his concern for his wife, even though he was a seriously ill patient.

During the summer the hospital had taken careful stock of the first wave experience of Covid-19 infections and Olive had reminded colleagues that the care commitment was to a relative as well as the patient. If relatives couldn't visit the patient, then it would be helpful to provide them with daily updates on care. In the first wave the hospital had been inundated with telephone enquiries to the different wards, at varying times of day and night, and this meant that nursing staff were distracted from their care-giving duties. At first, a protocol was agreed relating to who might be allowed to telephone in with enquiries. Then, however, Olive and colleagues had pressed for a family officer linked to the ward who would provide a once-daily bulletin of patient progress at an agreed time of the day. The hospital staff would ring out rather than relatives ring in. Nurses would of course personally telephone patients' spouses if the patient's condition worsened, but more routine bulletins would be provided by family officers (two retired nurses who were happy to volunteer help one step back from bedside care).

Olive described this to me as a logistical communication measure, but I ventured the possibility that it contributed as well to rapport building. If the patient became more severely ill, or was sedated, then they might still be assured that a loved one received updates. I asked Olive what this meant as regards the things she asked Abraham about. She explained that she always enquired about what the couple had discussed regarding Covid illness and especially about any particular worries that they had. The focus of needs and concerns varied between couples, but noting this down and having it attended to as a focus in daily briefings seemed very important.

'What were those as regards Abraham and Lillian?' I asked.

Olive answered:

Abraham and Lillian worried that if he survived, his cigarette-affected lungs might take a long time to improve. He saw himself as Lillian's carer and he didn't want to let her down. So, he wanted us to tell Lillian honestly about the state of his lungs and especially about any improvement. That seems odd given that his life was threatened, but their life signature was all about compensating for each other's difficulties.

I asked her if she passed on that detail to the ICU staff when they took over Abraham's care. Olive explained that she had written it down on Abraham's standard care plan. There was a place there for 'personal needs'. The ICU department also had a family officer, a very busy one, and when I checked with her too, she confirmed that her briefings to Lillian always included reference to Abraham's chest X-rays and any other results that lung function was improving. Whilst she could not promise a full recovery, the focus of concern was carried through, until Abraham emerged from the ICU and into the care of another nurse, called Joan, in the recovery ward.

What do you conclude from the above account of care continuity and liaison with relatives such as Lillian? Do you think that this is part of listening and rapport building? What does it tell you about the delivery of person-centred care – is it delivered by nurses or can it be provided through a wider system of care?

An outline answer is given at the end of this chapter.

The second period of more substantial rapport building with Abraham was delivered by Joan in the recovery ward. A native Londoner, she was proud of the efforts made to get patients home to their families once they had recovered and seemed sufficiently stable. Joan's background was in cardiac nursing and she had spent some time helping patients to rehabilitate after heart valve or coronary artery bypass surgery. In that setting patients had longer to recuperate, but there were still similarities between Covid and heart surgery recovery. Both required a progressive regime of physiotherapy that reduced the risks of immobilisation and helped develop the confidence of patients about what their bodies could do. The time available for recovery and rehabilitation on her ward now was very limited. The pressure to release bed spaces was relentless and patients in any case were usually keen to leave a worrying hospital environment. Patients were, however, also frightened that their condition might suddenly relapse as well.

Joan was reasonably practised in exploring the patient's narrative with them because this was a locally used approach in coronary rehabilitation as well. She explained that Hansen et al. (2016) had reported a narrative analysis approach based on linguistics (Griemas, 1983), and this described six care narrative factors that had to be understood through nurse enquiry:

- *The subject* (this is the patient and how they see their situation).
- *The object* (this was the goal to which individuals worked, the task that had to be completed. The problem was that the patient's goal and that of the hospital might not always coincide. Patients might prefer simply to rest, but tissue perfusion with oxygen was key to the avoidance of complications and that meant graduated mobilising. It was critical then to understand what motivated the patient).
- *The opponent* (this was anything that hindered or obstructed work towards an agreed goal. With the Covid-19 patients Joan encountered, this was often linked to fear that rehabilitation might cause a sudden collapse).
- *The helper* (this was anything or any person that helped the patient overcome barriers to an agreed goal, to becoming whole again. Joan was able to call on two physiotherapists who had also practised helping heart surgery patients and both understood how cautious patients might feel about exercises).
- *The giver* (this referred to the person who delivered care, who provided important information. Joan explained that patients usually assumed that the nurse was

the giver, but that sometimes it was possible to help the patient realise that they contributed work to the plan as well).

- *The receiver* (the person being assisted. Usually this was the patient but sometimes a relative might be the receiver – the nurse helping the relative to in turn help the patient).

I asked Joan whether this narrative analysis approach helped to shape the way she asked questions of a patient like Abraham. She explained:

> *It's not simply being nice, showing that you care. You see, if I don't understand what state Abraham was in coming off the ventilator, then I couldn't be sure how fast and hard I could press his mobilisation. I needed to understand how big a task he thought recuperation was. On this ward there is a huge variation in the extent to which patients become mobile before they go home to make room for other patients. It would be unwise to push all the patients at the same speed. Patients vary in their level of confidence and of course they had varying ideas about their state of health before they became ill. Certain safety-related goals, like climbing stairs if they have them at home, have to be met, but the plans are all very individual. The approach has to be adequately personal; this is not a rehabilitation boot camp.*

Practice tip

Don't be afraid to check how patients conceive of things, so that you can appreciate the risk, effort or commitment required. Rehabilitation, for instance, is a word that is clearly defined for most nurses but may evoke very different ideas for patients.

Activity 3.4   Critical thinking

Look back now at the narrative analysis framework that Joan used and decide for yourself whether you think it might be valuable.

- Could questions about the patient's feelings of readiness and their past and current health serve both a caring and a medical problem-solving purpose?
- What about words such as 'opponent' – does that help you to explore what might seem like barriers to nurses and patients beginning to explore and action a plan of care?

An outline answer is given at the end of this chapter.

Joan started with very open questions. She didn't ask Abraham, 'how do you see yourself now, as a subject?' That would have seemed strange. Instead, she asked questions such as 'how do you feel now?' and 'how does that compare with how you felt about your health before you became ill?' These are questions about the subject nonetheless. Her questions about the object were framed in a similar open way. 'Now that you're recovering, what would you like to achieve?' or 'what does getting better mean for you now?' Information about the opponent, the helper and the giver, in Joan's experience, usually come out of what the patient offers in response to the earlier questions. The patient describes their attitudes towards recovery and rehabilitation and indicates what roles they assume that they and others play.

Table 3.1 summarises Abraham's responses to Joan's gentle enquiries.

Table 3.1   Abraham's perceptions of circumstances

Narrative focus	Abraham's perceived circumstances
Subject	Abraham felt damaged by the virus, which left him feeling fatigued and vulnerable. He was uncertain about his resource of health, which he described in terms of energy and confidence. Both were important, he thought, if he was to get better and look after Lillian again. Just how damaged he was remained unclear to him.
Object	Abraham wanted to become fit again and by this he meant to overcome his breathlessness and fatigue. He wanted to avoid a relapse and had heard that this could happen with Covid-19 infections.
Opponent	Abraham accepted that fear might obstruct his progress; this related to the completion of mobility exercises. But fear could motivate too. He appreciated that obesity was a health risk. 'I've had a jolt', he said, 'this virus nearly killed me. But I'm still here'.
Helper	Abraham wanted a lot of information, about his illness, about long-term recovery, about getting better after being on a ventilator. But he wanted to listen and learn before he started doing a lot of physiotherapy. This would prove a tension as staff hoped to mobilise him relatively quickly.
Giver	Abraham saw Joan and colleagues as teachers rather than coaches. He thought that they were briefing him for things to do after his stay in hospital. He felt that he would help himself more later on, when he was able to 'get about again'. Abraham was disinclined to 'overdo' the mobilisation exercise work now and he hoped that Joan's teaching could be used at home when he felt less tired.
Receiver	Abraham saw himself as a learner, ready to understand. That didn't seem easy, though, as he struggled to concentrate. His mind felt 'foggy'. He didn't anticipate challenging himself, testing exercise boundaries; he felt very cautious.

Negotiating person-centred care (planning)

Looking back at Table 3.1, you may reasonably have concluded that there are both positives and negatives here. Abraham was certainly relieved to have survived his illness and felt ready to learn, but his perception of recuperation was a passive one.

He imagined his strength returning gradually and his confidence to test out that strength returning slowly too. The challenge is that the medical problem and his personal problem are not the same. The healthcare team need to prompt him on to explore as much activity as seems possible, provided that his observations remain stable and his blood oxygen saturation levels remain 90–93% at minimum. Joan and colleagues needed to counter the risks of immobility, especially after time spent on a ventilator. Patients recovering after artificial ventilation could sometimes suffer from a form of post-traumatic stress disorder, and Joan believed that focusing on a carefully managed exercise programme was a useful antidote to that risk (Garrouste-Orgeas et al., 2019). The clinical parameters as regards what represents safe rehabilitation are not the same as the confidence parameters of the patient. Joan's appraisal of what was safe was informed by her knowledge of immobility and recovery, whilst Abraham's notion of safety was bounded by fatigue and fear of what might happen if he mobilised quickly.

To reinforce this rather slow and feel-safe approach to rehabilitation, Abraham conceived of Joan as a teacher, when in practice she believed that she must coach Abraham through a series of graduated and carefully calibrated exercises, designed to enable him to become as mobile as possible. Complications of immobility, and the risks of further hospital-acquired infections, prompted Joan to try and enable Abraham to return home as soon as seemed safe. As was explained in Chapter 2, there is a need to help the patient with an understanding of the medical problem, the risks that they face, and to develop confidence that they can do something about this. Until Abraham has a sense of control, a feeling that he can act with minimum risk of further harm, he will not exercise very well. It seemed imperative to Joan that she help Abraham experiment with incremental mobility steps that would secure both independence and the ability to support Lillian again.

In Chapter 2 we learned that the negotiation of care and the planning of action might involve some difficult truths. The patient has sometimes to be confronted with issues that demand action. At the same time, however, it is necessary to sustain the patient's trust in our support, and to promote hope that they can succeed. Joan explained it this way:

Abraham started to frame his situation as one of learning and hiding. He felt that the more he learned, the more he might achieve in the future. However, he missed the point that knowledge wasn't enough. If he didn't try things out for himself, then he would never build confidence to work at his mobility exercises. Physio couldn't remain passive with staff putting his joints through a range of movements as they did in ICU. Abraham needed to test out mobilising, to check out tiredness and recovery from tiredness just like patients on a cardiac ward. He needed to feel reassured that we wouldn't push him recklessly, that we would monitor him carefully. I wouldn't simply tell him things, I would show him things, help him to explore a little more each day. Because of Covid restrictions there was little physio and occupational therapy support when he got home, so he would have to learn the basics in hospital.

Activity 3.5   Reflection

Reflect now on whether, in your experience, either you or a practice supervisor have taken such a firm stance with a patient as regards the role that the nurse would fulfil. In your experience, was the adoption of such a role successful or counter-productive then? In Abraham's case there seems little scope for a slower rehabilitation. The circumstances of the pandemic make it imperative that patients are discharged from hospital as soon as it's safe to do so. Did you or your practice supervisor argue the case for using a more robust stance, asking a patient to share responsibilities early on?

As this activity is based on your own reflection, no outline answer is provided at the end of the chapter.

I asked Joan what she then negotiated as goals and activities within the jointly agreed plan of care (see Table 3.2). I asked whether there was an element of 'tough love' associated with the recommended plan of care.

Table 3.2   Summary points from Abraham's care plan

Goal	Activity	Rationale
Safely discover how safe it is to mobilise, recovering activity, from before I became ill.	Complete incremental activities each day, walking, eating, shifting position, but checking each time how that felt and what if any consequences followed.	I need to feel safe but to realise where progress has been achieved. I feel very tired so exercising little and often should help build up my strength and confidence.
Manage my own progress, record what I achieve each day and how that links to any tests they do for me.	Fill in my own record and review what the staff add to that with blood and other tests. Use a scoring system that rates my level of breathlessness before and after every mobilising session.	I get to feel a sense of control. I can tell Lillian what I have managed over time. I won't get pushed along beyond what feels safe to me.
Keep in daily contact with Lillian.	Daily video call to reassure Lillian that all is well. I can learn about how she has been coping too.	We hope that Lillian can help you sustain your physiotherapy work too, Abraham (Joan).

Joan negotiated three care goals with Abraham, arguing that limiting the number would help concentrate their work and make it easier for him to sense progress. The first goal was for Abraham to discover how it felt to mobilise again. Joan explained that patients feared taking big strides, but that she explained that to sit still might be to slip backwards. Not only might Abraham run the risk of hospital-acquired infections whilst weak, but he would not feel confident acting as a support to Lillian later. She explained to Abraham that she could not promise a resolution of fatigue but that she believed that patients who worked effectively earlier on in recovery suffered the fewest residual problems with Covid later. She asked him to explore how it felt to mobilise rather than set a number of steps or exercise repetitions a day. Abraham felt cautious about her claim that early mobilising patients did better later on.

You believe that? challenged Abraham, You don't know they do better for sure?

No, I don't know it for sure, the research isn't done yet, Joan responded. But I believe that it's true from the work I used to do with patients who had heart problems. They were frightened as well, and there the patients who exercised the heart … got the better results. You are exercising your lungs, getting more oxygen around your body. I think your thinking will seem less foggy if you do that. I think that you will boost your morale if you find you can do more than you imagined.

The second goal was for Abraham to manage his own progress record – that which included details of his blood oxygen levels, blood pressure, pulse and respiration rate (breaths per minute), and his own notes about levels of breathlessness and fatigue. Abraham would score each out of 5, where 5 meant that he experienced no difficulties (best score) and 0 represented very significant difficulties (worst score). Abraham would have the chance to discuss his record with the medical consultant each day and to add notes before and after exercise.

You're giving me a sense of control, observed Abraham. But you're not letting me sit this out, are you.

Joan answered:

You need to get oxygen around your body, to improve your lungs and to feel strong again. Anxiety-provoking as exercise is, you will get better if you attempt that. You can't afford to sit this out, Abraham.

The third agreed goal was to keep Lillian abreast of his progress daily using a video call on an electronic tablet that the ward had purchased just for such purpose. Joan had established that Lillian was used to such calls as she regularly called her sister using Skype.

That's something that I want most of all, said Abraham. Bulletins aren't the same anymore. Is that a carrot, though? I only get the call if I exercise?

Joan assured him no. Lillian needed the call and Abraham could show her his walking exercise, the physiotherapist or herself holding the mobile phone steady.

Activity 3.6   Critical thinking

Answer the following questions now about Joan's care planning with Abraham:

1. Why does Joan lay such emphasis on exploring how it feels to mobilise each day?
2. What is the value of asking Abraham to control his own monitoring records?
3. Joan suggested that Abraham score dyspnoea/fatigue difficulties on a scale of 0–5 with 5 representing the best score each time. That's the reverse of scoring that you might see, for example, on a pain chart. Why do you think she arranged the record that way?
4. Why do you think that Lillian plays such an important role in the care plan?

An outline answer is given at the end of this chapter.

Practice tip

It's a good idea to write many of the care plan items in terms of what the patient aims for and achieves (use of 'I'). This helps engage the patient in planning and assures them that we remain interested in their perspective. Activities could detail the repetition of daily nurse work, but that becomes a performance log for nurses. It is valuable to acknowledge that such may vary and is negotiated. A rationale column is a good idea and there is no reason why both the patient and the nurse should not add entries to this. Rationale helps clarify ongoing narratives of care.

Collaborating on person-centred care (implementing)

In Chapter 2 we learned that collaboration in person-centred care is channelled through the adoption of roles, through monitoring of progress and perhaps the identification of additional care goals or the adjustment of existing ones. In Abraham's case, Joan adopted the role of personal coach. There were, of course, other patients with pressing needs, but when Joan was not able to personally superintend his carefully graded mobility exercises three times a day, then one or other of the two physiotherapists would. The mobility exercises included not only the safe transfer from bed to chair and from chair to an upright stance, but a carefully measured series of short walks designed to help Abraham judge what seemed possible. Patients who rehabilitate after mechanical ventilation, those who have struggled with breathing, are often initially challenged by giddiness, postural hypotension and weakness as they move from horizontal to upright (Hashem et al., 2016). Proprioception – that is, the sense of your body within space; necessary, for instance, to lower yourself into a chair – can be badly affected.

On the ward other patients were also completing mobilisation exercises and I asked Joan whether she thought that this encouraged patients or whether it might seem a daunting training regime. Joan explained that all the patients' mobilisation programmes were individualised, based upon the patient's age, previous levels of mobility, baseline observations, tolerance of fatigue and dyspnoea. Those unable to mobilise a great deal were still able to complete deep breathing exercises that helped to counter the areas of lung consolidation that the virus and inflammation had produced. Oxygen was used to prepare for mobility exercises and available again for support immediately afterwards. Whilst some patients mobilised with the help of a mobile oxygen cylinder, it was important for the patients to realise that they could incrementally complete short activities without oxygen canula in situ. Abraham watched the others as they progressed and after three days' care he observed that several other patients were managing to mobilise rather well. This encouraged him.

What in Joan's view remained critical about the mobility programme was that it was carefully matched against patient observations. It was critical to check that baseline observations such as pulse oximetry (blood oxygen saturation levels) remained within safe limits – that blood pressure did not suddenly drop or respiratory rate soar. Not only might the patient then collapse, but other patients would be daunted because the staff had pressed the exercise too hard. She explained that Abraham and his colleagues were assessed daily, and that the review included not only respiratory function, but also whether the patients were well hydrated, eating well, whether they had secured a good night's sleep and whether their morale that morning seemed upbeat.

I want now to focus upon Abraham's self-monitoring of his mobility progress, because this offers several points about person-centred care. In Part 1 it was emphasised that such care is heavily reliant upon acknowledging and managing patient perceptions. The case was made that perceptions might tell us about their values, attitude, motivation, fears and needs. Now, though, the importance of perceptions is taken further because the approach that Joan used makes use of feedback mechanisms familiar in cognitive behaviour therapy and which highlight why the person-centred care approach can be so powerful (e.g. Lindgreen et al., 2016).

Before Abraham commenced each exercise session, he was encouraged to prepare by rehearsing his purpose for the programme (getting fit to help Lillian) and to note down his baseline observations. Joan emphasised that the short walk was not a race; he could draw breath, pausing as he wished. She would be there to support his arm. He was encouraged to rehearse aloud (in short commentary) how his breathing felt as he moved, and where any fatigue seemed to affect him the most. Abraham reported that his legs felt very heavy and cumbersome. He didn't feel that he made them move smoothly. Joan and Abraham commenced their walks, aiming for a view from the ward's sitting-room windows. The view of the garden was a 'halfway house' reward. Abraham could start his walks from progressively further points from the window, rising from an anchored wheelchair.

In cognitive behavioural therapy the patient regularly attends to the experience of the phenomenon (in this case gentle, supported walking), notes feelings evoked and applies meanings to it (Kazantzis et al., 2017). Such meanings may be negative or positive (e.g. this is exhausting, or I'm doing well). Attention focuses on discrete experiences: those that may have seemed barriers at the start. So in Abraham's case he was encouraged to attend to his breathing. Did it seem harder or easier, did it seem noisier? What did Abraham notice if he walked a little more upright, did that seem to make breathing easier? What happened to Abraham's sense of balance if he tried to walk less stooped forward? As Abraham noted each experience and added a perception, feeling and meaning to the experience, Joan explained measures that could be used to counter the anxiety that resulted (see Figure 3.1 for an overview of Joan's work). Why not pause now? Concentrate on slower and deeper breaths, that might make your chest feel a bit more uncomfortable, but do you see how the feeling of giddiness or nausea reduces? Helping the patient back and forth, between their experiences and what might counter worries, is a feedback mechanism in action. Joan assisted Abraham to explore how much he could modify the barriers to his progress and how he could explore incrementally greater achievements that worked towards the goal of going home to Lillian.

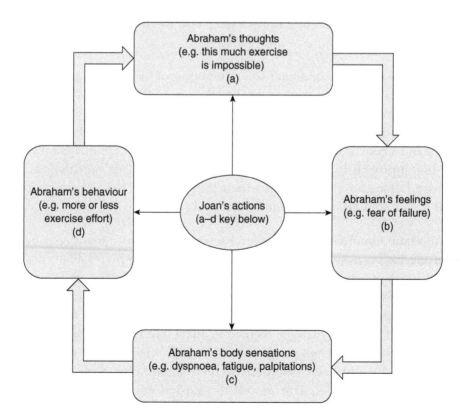

Figure 3.1   Cognitive behavioural cycle and Joan's intervention

Key for Figure 3.1

a.   Joan helps Abraham understand why he thinks of himself as vulnerable, but helps him remember what he was capable of before. They observe the progress of others and she sets up a progress record that he can check back on. She explains the importance of improving his circulation, the oxygen benefits that it brings.

b.   She helps him review his feelings that he cannot recover because of fatigue and fear of failure. She explains that by monitoring his progress in small steps, that fear can be countered. He is in control and can utilise oxygen supply as needed.

c.   She uses the progress record to help him monitor improvements in dyspnoea and to prove to him that baseline observations remain stable or improve. Joan helps Abraham review his sensations in a new way.

d.   Using oxygen, targets for exercise, she gradually helps him extend his walking range (behaviour). Joan taught Abraham how to interpret his blood oxygen saturation levels so he could identify improvements and what was secure and stable. Abraham is encouraged to review his successes so that he can think differently about his abilities.

Activity 3.7   Reflection

Do you remember any clinical experiences where you made use of cognitive behavioural feedback activity, such as that deployed with Abraham? For example, have you helped a patient overcome a panic attack, or perhaps deal with a phobia? Have you helped them reimagine what it means to receive chemotherapy for cancer? Jot your example down.

Cognitive behavioural therapy is firmly a psychological strategy, expertly utilised by advanced practitioners and therapists, but it is too, in simple form, something that registered nurses regularly use to help patients direct their perceptions to best purpose. To return to the narrative analysis framework suggested by Hansen et al. (2016), it can help the patient to think of themselves as a giver as well as a receiver. It can help the patient to develop greater confidence after a time of feeling extremely vulnerable.

As this activity is based on your own reflection, no outline answer is given at the end of the chapter.

I asked Joan to reflect on her mobilisation work with Abraham, focusing in particular on his perceptions and whether that seemed to help him gently progress with the series of exercises. As you will see below, it wasn't a straightforward process and she needed to draw on her experience as regards how best to help him.

After each of the graded walks taken Abraham reconnected up to his oxygen supply and we allocated 10 minutes for him to recompose himself. I always encouraged him, though, to take his own pulse every couple of minutes, noting how it slowed down at rest. I encouraged him to note the slowing rate of his breathing and how much less laboured it seemed. Then we would debrief about the experience. I know that sounds grand, a rather military thing, but it was really a conversation in which he evaluated what the walk had felt like. He said one day that he felt as though his heart was huge, that it pounded within his chest. To reassure Abraham, I used the stethoscope to listen to his chest, counted his pulse rate and measured his blood pressure. They were all safely within limits. That reassured him. Still, I made a note of the experience and checked with the doctor to see if any extra tests were needed.

Practice tip

Sometimes the briefest patient observations and reflections will tell you whether you are guiding and supporting them well. A thank you is obviously a recognition of your work, but so too might be expression of relief about threats abated, or small milestones achieved. Spot the indicators; savour the insights.

Evaluating person-centred care (evaluating)

In my experience the evaluation of agreed care is incompletely explored in some care settings. Nurses and patients may simply be content that care has seemed uneventful. The judgement on care seems stark; it is simply about whether care failed. If significant problems arose, then evaluation might be extensive; perhaps a complaint might be lodged and answered. When problems arise, causation is explored. In uneventful care, however, evaluation is sometimes neglected. There is rarely analysis of why something seemed to work especially well. In person-centred nursing care, though, evaluation is important for two key reasons. First, the nurse wishes to learn whether the individual care measures agreed have worked. Future goal setting may rest on determining what is realistic or most effective. Was the care outcome something that was anticipated, was it better or worse than was hoped for? Perhaps the result of care was something unex-pected, something discovered through serendipity. Second, though, the nurse wants to know what the patient thinks about their own part in the proceedings. In most instances person-centred care involves liaison, and that might offer insights into the functioning of healthcare as a service too. Person-centred care has the potential to energise a patient, to build confidence because they have been asked to partner the nurse in care. That seemed especially important with Abraham because at stake was his level of confidence in not only going home, but also caring for his wife. Two relatively immobile people in a household might face additional problems in the future.

Abraham and Joan sat down to review the nursing care on the evening before his dis-charge from hospital. He was now able to mobilise briefly without oxygen and, whilst he remained very tired, he agreed that he had made significant improvements during his stay on the recovery ward. The walking exercises, rising from and sitting back into chairs, had been important work, improving his stamina, but they had also helped him to believe that he could slowly manage the stairs up to their bedroom at home. Abraham thought he would manage to take baths, to dress and undress. Abraham was confident that he could balance himself well.

> *I don't feel apprehensive, said Abraham, though when we started with the exercises, I would never have believed that I would climb those steps. I imagined myself sleeping on the sofa in the living room …*

Joan asked him what he felt about being urged to exercise, rather than to listen to instruction about it. Was that a good thing, or did he now leave the ward feeling that the staff had pressed him too hard? Abraham responded that he had found the walking quite tough. He didn't believe that he was as strong as Joan thought he was. However, if he didn't test out the exercise, then it might seem no easier to begin it later at home, where nurses and therapists weren't on hand to help. Abraham said that he would feel a little more confident to carry on making some changes after his narrow escape from death. He would reduce his body weight by a couple of stone. He conceded that he had become too sedentary and his body weight had made the physiotherapy that much harder. Joan cautioned that post his illness, problems could still remain, although she suspected that patients who managed more exercise improved their chances of a complete recovery.

What didn't go so well? Joan asked, returning to her open question strategy. Note the wording of that. She didn't ask *what did we let you down on?* or *what weren't you able to contribute?* Open questions such as these enable the patient to frame evaluation in their own terms and signal useful information about what the patient values most.

Abraham paused. His daily video chat with Lillian hadn't worked as he'd imagined it might. Whilst his wife had greatly encouraged his mobility exercises, she had started to use the video conversations to quiz Joan and her colleagues about recovery from mechanical ventilation. It had become apparent to both Abraham and Joan that Lillian was very anxious about what mechanical ventilation might do to a patient.

You explained things well, said Abraham. *Lillian seemed to understand by the end, but I hadn't anticipated that she would fret like that.*

Activity 3.8   Critical thinking

Pause now to think about Lillian's anxieties and what you have read above about taking roles during care collaboration. Do you think that Joan perhaps missed a point when she arranged for Lillian to help motivate Abraham during his walking exercises?

An outline answer is given at the end of this chapter.

Abraham had a question for Joan after they had worked through a review of the agreed care goals and decided that they had been successfully achieved.

> *Would you have used the same approach with me if the hospital hadn't needed the beds so badly?*

Joan smiled. It was a good question.

> *When I prompted you to go on lengthening the walks those last days, I was always taking your pulse, listening to your breathing, wasn't I,* she observed. *I knew what should be possible, I've seen your X-rays, read your charts. But I didn't want you to despair and blow up at me.*

> *Wouldn't do that, you're only trying to help,* insisted Abraham quickly.

> *But do you see … you can't measure confidence so easily on the chart. You wrote down how tired you were, whether you felt relieved to have met a milestone, but I don't know how well you cope. I didn't know how much adversity you have overcome in the past,* said Joan.

> *I suppose not,* agreed Abraham, *you didn't ask me if I stuck at projects.*

> Joan smiled. *If I'd asked you or Lillian about that, I would have helped you with a little more confidence, wouldn't I?*

> *You did splendidly nurse, just fine,* insisted Abraham.

> *And you did as well,* said Joan.

Activity 3.9   Reflection

Reading this summary of Abraham's care, what do you now think evaluation is really about in person-centred care? Is it, for example, about performance, who fulfilled their role well? Or is it instead about learning and a recognition of what insights amount to? Should evaluation acknowledge work yet to be done, commenting on the extent of progress? Jot an idea or two down before looking at my suggestions.

An outline answer is given at the end of this chapter.

Case study insights

This case study was chosen to help you formulate an overview of person-centred care in action. Pandemic circumstances taxed the nurses' ability to deliver ideal person-centred care to Abraham, both because he was at first too ill to partner Olive in care planning and because the sheer volume of care demands forced nurses to determine what could be equitably offered to the patient group as a whole. It is not necessarily possible to make person-centred care all-encompassing – an approach viable in every circumstance. This case study illustrates where person-centred care made the clearest contribution. Person-centred care is most readily expressed as a form of psychological support. In the ICU the nurse talks to the unconscious patient, addressing him by name. It is unclear what the patient can hear. But the greatest chance to personalised care occurs elsewhere, before and after time spent on a mechanical ventilator. Discussion of Abraham's care has centred on passages of interaction where psychology and partnership had the biggest part to play.

What person-centred care can and cannot do is an important question because it relates to the different care approaches that you read about in Chapter 1. Standard care packages (in this instance linked to countering the medical risks of Covid-19) have a key part to play in nursing care. There is little scope for patients and nurses, for example, to debate the merits of ventilator support. Evidence (for example, associated with the risks of a cytokine storm) has a critical role to play as well. It would seem rather strange to discount such protocol or evidence-based advice, insisting instead that patient-expressed needs trump everything else. Sometimes the gravity of a medical problem (the risk to life from a virus) outweighs a personal problem and the search for more nuanced and attentive ways to agree care. Sometimes the role of person-centred care is to help the patient to understand the necessity of guidelines. As we will see in other case studies in this book, at other times person-centred care has the lead and choice expands.

The next insight that I hoped you gained was that it is unwise to think of person-centred care as a rigid, stage-bound formula. Abraham's hospital episode involved two stages of relationship building, the second of which was understandably more complete than the first. Patients enter a healthcare system to meet their needs and whilst every effort is made to communicate patient hopes and aspirations to colleagues as care proceeds, it is not necessarily possible to ensure that person-centred care is seamless. In healthcare there are challenges to joining up person-centred care as a staged process. In this instance, a medical emergency (failing respiration) intervened to halt a simple progression of the care relationship. Nonetheless, both Olive and Joan were sufficiently confident to personalise care within the bounds of circumstance. Both nurses had concern for the patient experience and both anticipated patient needs, working hard to help Abraham secure the best from the service available.

The third insight that I hope you will take away is that the nurses orchestrated the use of information, evidence and protocol, enabling Abraham to feel respected in the midst of the system. Did you notice how important it was for Olive to translate research evidence for Abraham and how necessary it was for Joan to gain Abraham's commitment to the recommended exercise approach? There was no set target of steps per day. Instead, Joan helped Abraham appreciate what he could safely achieve. Theory informed both her approach to narrative analysis and to the business of linking exercise to feelings and meanings, the better to realise what was possible (cognitive behavioural therapy). Excellent person-centred care is strategic and it is intelligent practice. The nurse makes use of what they know to lead the patient when they are in a vulnerable state.

Practice tip

If you work in a hard-pressed acute-care environment, remember that being person-centred can start from quite modest beginnings. Simply acknowledging what you have heard the patient say is a vital start. Recognising anxiety is an important matter, even if you cannot entirely remove it.

Chapter summary

Person-centred care may be harder to orchestrate in some acute-care settings, but opportunities to individualise care often increase as the patient progresses. Person-centred care is delivered by a series of clinicians so it's important to communicate well, building the theme of reassurance and support. In these settings, because partnered care can take time to grow, anticipation of commonly encountered needs becomes more important and the interpretation of evidence becomes a key skill. The story of Abraham shows how nurses can humanise an otherwise daunting environment and attend to the needs of a patient and his very important marital relationship.

Activities: Brief outline answers

Activity 3.1 Reflection (p48)

The medical problem is firmly about risks associated with deteriorating respiratory function, and possible damage to other organs of the body. It is concerned with cross-infection risks and problems that can arise when patients are managed on a ventilator. Covid-19 represents an assault on the body. But I think the personal problem builds out of the threat of that; it is concerned with patient anxiety and Abraham's circumstances of living. He feels responsible for his wife, but he doesn't understand the full extent of the risk before him. Does it matter that he was an asthmatic, for instance? Initially Abraham didn't know. Because Abraham fears hospital and infection there, he could make a serious mistake and demand care at home. The nature of the medical problem needs to be explained to him and why by taking risks associated with hospital admission he may yet secure a better outcome.

Activity 3.3 Reflection (p54)

I wonder if you were encouraged by this sort of hospital planning? The NHS has been battered by the pandemic, but it has worked with nurses such as Olive to see how systems could be adjusted to make the service seem both more workable and humane. Issuing progress bulletins could (in theory) be very impersonal, but if nurses feed the right sort of information to a family officer, then the update might seem very personal and supportive indeed. Bulletins rely on the nurses' understanding of patient anxieties and needs in the first instance. Arranged in that way, the service builds rapport with patient and relative. Classically, person-centred care is mediated by bedside staff, especially nurses, but I think that a service can be very person-centred as well.

Activity 3.4 Critical thinking (p55)

I think that mnemonics and other aide-memoires have a valuable part to play in person-centred nursing care. But be careful about turning them into rigid prescriptions for care. Frameworks are there to facilitate your practice. So in Hansen et al.'s (2016) reported framework, you might con-sider adjusting the words a little. The 'receiver' is nearly always the patient or relative, so you might simply designate that. Perhaps 'barriers' seems a better word than 'opponent' when describing what might hamper care. I might use 'objective' rather than 'object' to describe the purpose of care. You are allowed to do this – carefully examining what makes a framework easier to operate.

What I like about the framework is that it focuses on relationship building (signalling our inter-est in what worries the patient) but also focuses attention on the clinical need, the work ahead. In this sense the framework is strategic. You are not simply asking questions to express a concern for the patient; you are identifying that which might help solve a problem before you.

Activity 3.6 Critical thinking (p60)

Here are my answers to the questions.

1. Joan wishes to convey several things taking this approach. First, that the rehabilitation programme has scope to accommodate what Abraham feels, what seems possible to him. It is a personal recovery contract between them. Second, she wants to use an understanding of experiences and feelings to help Abraham realise what progress means. If Joan doesn't encourage Abraham to record such thoughts, it might be harder for him to review progress or problems over the coming days. At minimum Joan signals that she is concerned about Abraham's feelings, the apprehension that he experiences.

2. If Abraham manages his own monitoring records, he gains a greater sense of control. He can check his own results at any time and ask questions about them. There is much less chance then that a patient fears that information is being held back from them. The increased sense of control that Abraham secures might help him to commit all the more to the rehabilitation effort.

3. Joan told me that the scoring system is a positive one. The higher the score, the better the achievement, and this is what people are more accustomed to when rating products, services or performances. That might help motivate Abraham, even if he is doing his own scoring. This seems to me an excellent idea; it works with the patient's experience of scoring things elsewhere.

4. Lillian is both a focus of Abraham's concerns and a likely resource. A loved partner is well placed to motivate a patient in completing rehabilitation exercises.

Activity 3.8 Critical thinking (p65)

I wonder if you spotted that Joan has thought of Lillian as a fellow carer when in fact she is also another potential casualty of the Covid-19 infection? Whilst nurses hope to work constructively with relatives to advance person-centred care, it is necessary to assess what the relative can offer. How confident was Lillian to promote the mobility exercises? Were there questions about Covid-19, about hospital and recovery from illness, that Joan might have anticipated before Lillian was recruited as an accomplice? We might assume that a relative wants to help, but it is also possible to overestimate their capacity to assist, or perhaps their readiness to play a particular role.

Activity 3.9 Reflection (p66)

I would encourage you to think of person-centred nursing care evaluation as fulfilling multi-ple functions. It should certainly include elements of performance judgement: what worked well and what seemed poor or incomplete. We must not shy away from criticism. But it is quintessentially, too, a review of learning. If person-centred care is about negotiating care, about teamwork and responding sensitively to patient needs, then we must examine how easy that was and what measures seemed to assist with the process. Notice how much Joan transfers from coronary care rehabilitation where she previously worked. This was only possible because she speculated about the extent to which cardiac- and Covid-19-challenged patients might have needs in common. What can be liberating about person-centred care evaluation is that it is not entirely focused on service provision, and our performance as a nurse. It is easier and less threatening to evaluate what 'we' did; what we learned en route. Person-centred care has the potential to substantially improve nursing practice because of this, making practice a little less defensive, a little more explorative.

Further reading

Francis, G (2021) *Intensive Care: A GP, a Community and Covid-19.* London: Profile Press/ Welcome Collection.

Gavin Francis offers a diary of what he terms the 'plague year' (2020). Even though you may have studied/practised in the midst of this, it is instructive to look back and take stock of how it made you think about your work and what seemed possible to contract as care with patients. Covid-19 radically reshaped care priorities and challenged clinicians to re-evaluate their purpose and role.

Macciochi, J (2020) *Immunity: The Science of Staying Well.* London: Thorsons (Harper Collins).

This book is written for the general public; as the pandemic swept across the globe, there came a growing public demand for guidance on how to boost the immune system and stay well. In anticipation of the many questions that you may still be asked, I recommend this accessible book. As well as examining the guidance offered here, it is worth reflecting on the language and explanations used. What might you take from this regarding how best to make information usable for patients?

Rogers, J and Maini, A (2016) *Coaching for Health: Why It Works and How to Do It.* Maidenhead: Open University Press.

This would be my must-read textbook if you were inspired by Joan's work with Abraham in this case study. It's an upbeat explanation of what coaching is and how it can enrich a great deal of healthcare that we call person-centred. Make no mistake, coaching requires resource, especially of time with a patient or patient group, but if you are interested in patient rehabilitation in a person-centred way, then this text will carry you forward.

Useful websites

Visit **www.youtube.com** and search for the following video: 'A COVID-19 Survivor's Story', produced in November 2020 by CoxHealth, Springfield, USA.

This brief video summarises the sudden and daunting illness of Mike Hemphill who contracted Covid-19, as seen from the point of view of his daughters in particular. The video offers a family perspective of the assault of the virus and what it meant to those affected. Fear and anxiety you might anticipate, but I think it's worth noting the way the episode is narrated. Notice the importance of time; the speed of illness onset. Notice the way in which Mike characterises recovery in terms of learning. Mike's daughter reminds us that Covid affects older people, and Mike is not (as she sees him) an old person, but the challenge of learning to walk again represents a major challenge. Notice how closely the narratives of patient and family interlace.

Visit **www.youtube.com** and search for the following videos:

Vanessa May: Narrative analysis. Manchester University.

Graham Gibbs: The analysis of narratives. University of Huddersfield.

These two YouTube videos, filmed lectures by social scientists, offer further explanations of narratives (stories) and how they operate. Don't worry that these apply to social science research; the focus on narratives is much the same – a quest to understand experience and ascribed meanings by the storyteller. Notice how in these accounts narrative can take different forms (e.g. spoken, written, even action). It is worth remembering that the individual who stories their experience may be discovering things as they go or they may reinforce a stance that they take, narrating why it is defensible. We turn to a more leisurely opportunity to understand a patient narrative in the next case study (Chapter 4).

Chapter 4 Case study two

Helping John cope with surgery

NMC Future Nurse Standards of Proficiency for Registered Nurses

This chapter will address the following platforms and proficiencies:

Platform 1: Being an accountable professional

At the point of registration, the registered nurse will be able to:

1.8 demonstrate the knowledge, skills and ability to think critically when applying evidence and drawing on experience to make evidence-informed decisions in all situations.

1.9 understand the need to base all decisions regarding care and interventions on people's needs and preferences, recognising and addressing any personal and external factors that may unduly influence your decisions.

1.11 communicate effectively using a range of skills and strategies with colleagues and people at all stages of life and with a range of mental, physical, cognitive and behavioural health challenges.

Platform 2: Promoting health and preventing ill health

At the point of registration, the registered nurse will be able to:

2.9 use appropriate communication skills and strength-based approaches to support and enable people to make informed choices about their care to manage health challenges in order to have satisfying and fulfilling lives within the limitations caused by reduced capability, ill health and disability.

Platform 3: Assessing needs and planning care

At the point of registration, the registered nurse will be able to:

3.4 understand and apply a person-centred approach to nursing care, demonstrating shared assessment, planning, decision making and goal setting when working with people, their families, communities and populations of all ages.

Platform 4: Providing and evaluating care

At the point of registration, the registered nurse will be able to:

4.2   work in partnership with people to encourage shared decision making, in order to support individuals, their families and carers to manage their own care when appropriate.

Chapter aims

After reading this chapter, you will be able to:

* understand the ways in which an anxious patient might be prepared for planned surgery in a person-centred way;
* demonstrate the way in which different healthcare professionals can work together using evidence, experience and patient insight to anticipate risks and negotiate a best way forward.

Explanatory note

In this case study, John is described as the service user when referring to his life in the residential community and as the patient when dealing with the hospital, this reflecting terminology norms in each location.

Introduction

In the last case study we explored aspects of person-centred care where healthcare services were under considerable duress and where the patient was less well equipped to negotiate person-centred care. In this next case study, about John, the healthcare context is less pressurised but the challenges of sensitively partnering the patient in care remain. Patients dealing with a learning disability have very individual needs when confronted with sudden change and they need assistance to transition from a well-known daily routine through something as threatening as surgery and back to a sense of security (Painter et al., 2018). The case study highlights the need to understand the patient's perceptions of change (e.g. diagnosis of bowel cancer, recommended surgery and admission to hospital) and to access the narrative that the patient runs about what is happening to them. But the case study also highlights the importance of arranging collaborative care, one that draws on expertise from several different sources. Those who know a great deal about the patient are every bit as important as those who know more about cancer and the best treatment regimen. This case study helps you to connect up narrative analysis with the creation of a safe care environment, one that enables the patient to complete a stay in hospital with a minimum of anxiety.

In this case study different care agencies played a role in the support of the patient. It was important to keep a careful check on what the care support team was trying to achieve. To do this they used a simple mnemonic (PERSON) to remind them of person-centred care precepts that they were following (Toluwalese et al., 2019).

Perception: In person-centred care it is important at all stages to understand and respect the perceptions of the patient – that relating not only to the change but regarding their daily life before as well. We can only understand the threat posed by an illness if we understand the scale and scope of mental adjustments necessary (Nunstedt et al., 2017). Change represents a threat, especially if it requires not only a change to daily activities of living but also a change in location.

Explore: Healthcare staff need to sensitively explore what the illness or injury and any treatment might mean for the person and their usual coping. If the patient has a limited adaptive capacity, then the change ahead must be modified as far as possible to help the patient keep threat within reasonable bounds. With a patient such as John, narrative analysis is a very important care skill, as is the strategic use of the person's known history provided by his carers.

Relate: In Part 1 of this book we highlighted how a medical problem (here it is bowel cancer) might collide with a personal problem (e.g. managing daily life in a secure manner). There is often an urgent need to proceed, reducing the risk of disease recurrence later. However, the patient needs adequate time to accommodate the risk before them. When patients suffer from a learning disability this cannot simply be managed through information giving. The patient needs to feel that the information giver has their best interests at heart, so the manner of interaction between patient and carers becomes important too.

Source: It can be tempting for healthcare professionals to see a treatment regime as relatively routine, as a familiar series of steps and measures which usually produces a safe and beneficial outcome. However, to be so complacent with a patient dealing with a learning disability would be unwise (Chinn and Homeyard, 2017). This is not simply another bowel resection operation, the formation of a temporary stoma and the usual recovery support post-anaesthetic. The possible sources of anxiety for a patient may extend much further. Hospital, for example, might seem significantly more threatening. Nurses must understand the source of patient needs and concerns.

Outline a plan: Notice the emphasis on outline. When we negotiate care and agree a plan, it is one that might have to change as events unfold and we better understand the patient's experiences. Where a patient deals with a learning disability it is important not only that proposed actions are clear and adequately understood, but also that the rationale for each is carefully rehearsed and checked.

Notify: Once the plan is agreed, we need to liaise with others to ensure that the plan can be actioned. This is not 'notify the patient' (they are a partner in care planning). We notify third parties of our intentions, the way we hope to proceed, and this accents the need for successful consultation with other resource providers.

Activity 4.1   Reflection

What do you think are the merits of the PERSON mnemonic, when planning person-centred care with a patient? Do you think it has advantages where patient perceptions play an especially large role?

An outline answer is given at the end of this chapter.

Case study: John

John is a 60-year-old single man who has, for the last 10 years, lived within a sheltered community supporting people with learning disabilities. John is of a cheerful disposition, but he is fearful of anything that disrupts his regular routine. Sudden change can cause him to become agitated and sometimes verbally aggressive.

As part of a screening programme, John was checked for abnormal cells or blood within the stool. The investigators called him to clinic with his regular support worker, Alice. Further investigations were carried out that Alice explained in terms of whether his gut was working well. John knew about guts as, when working at a hotel, he had cleaned rabbit carcasses in the kitchen. The doctor gently told him that he had a cancer of his gut, but that the tests revealed that it was limited to the muscle wall and that if a portion of his gut was cut out (a left hemicolectomy, technical terminology not used with John), then the disease could probably be taken away. The doctor explained that for a while he would have a 'bag on his belly' to collect the poo, but that, later, another operation would mean that he could use the toilet again in the normal way. It was possible to 'mend his gut' provided that he had an operation very soon.

Learning that he had cancer, and that he needed surgery, was a major change that John wasn't ready for. He needed to process the information a little at a time, so Alice arranged to rehearse this as three stories, (a) becoming ill, even though I don't feel poorly, (b) needing to go to hospital and have an operation, and then, (c) being different in the way that I go to the toilet. The days after John was advised of his illness, he became tearful and withdrawn and Alice noticed that he didn't want to eat with the others. John said that there was *something wrong inside me because of my eating and that it was best to eat alone in case others got sick.*

Anticipating patient care

The needs of people living with a learning disability are highly individual and they reflect not only their intellectual capacity but their living circumstances as well. Service users bring to care negotiation not only their problems reasoning, but also their experience of how others have responded to them in the past. A patient might have been abused earlier in their life; they may have been bullied or dismissed as beyond help and unworthy of opportunity. Such caveats noted, however, there are some frequently occurring features of the patient's needs that Alice and others were keenly aware of.

John, like the rest of us, formulates mental templates to help interpret the world about him. In a textbook on reasoning (Price, 2021), I explain how individuals develop more or less useful ways to reason day-to-day demands that seem beneficial and which are well received by others. People learn to conceptualise the world around them and what seems either threatening or comforting within that. Because no individual can expect to analyse in detail every moment-by-moment personal encounter, we develop a series of working templates: ways of conceiving of situations that seem more or less successful. Typically, in earlier years the working templates are less refined and that produces emotional problems as individuals confront more complex situations associated with growing up (e.g. sexual relationships). However, over time the young adult develops more nuanced ways of reasoning events and circumstances and this enables them to become more confident, adaptive individuals able to cope with a growing array of challenges in life.

In people with learning disabilities, however, the flexibility of mental templates used by an individual may be much more limited (Corbett, 2019). The individual copes by living in a rather more circumscribed way with a series of daily activities that not only help structure the day but also provide reassurance to the individual. The need to anticipate what might happen next is of paramount importance to an individual and if change is rapid and radical, then the individual may feel disorientated, anxious or even aggressive. The resource of emotional response to change might be severely limited.

Confronted with urgent change, the patient with a learning disability might:

- experience sudden and hard-to-control episodes of anxiety (Dagnan et al., 2018);
- try out other mental-template approaches used to cope with other events (e.g. aggression, withdrawal or pretending to understand) (Kiernan et al., 2019);
- concentrate on particular information and ignore other important explanations (resulting later in potential confusion and feelings of distrust);
- suddenly refuse to liaise with those assisting them. Crises of trust may quickly arise when events and requirements do not pan out as the patient anticipated.

Patients dealing with a learning disability are more likely to suffer from anxiety (Dagnan et al., 2018; Hermans et al., 2013). Those, for example, dealing with a condition within the autistic spectrum are especially prone to anxiety (Keefer et al., 2016). There is a need to enable the patient to rehearse what is going to happen, so that the strangeness of change is curtailed.

Practice tip

A useful exercise is to reflect on your own working templates, the way in which you explain common experiences to yourself, and the best ways to address those. Recognising more rigid working templates might alert you to situations where your care enquiry might seem less empathetic. We sometimes imagine that others cope just as we do.

Activity 4.2   Critical thinking

Imagine for a moment now that you have suddenly been asked to deliver a paper at a conference attended by several thousand people. How does this make you feel? What habitual ways of reasoning (templates) might you be able to draw upon to cope with this sudden challenge? Now look at the story of John above. What there suggests that John is searching for a new way to reason what is happening to him?

An outline answer is given at the end of this chapter.

Relating and person-centred care (assessing)

John's lead carer Alice anticipates just what time in hospital and surgery might entail for him. Not only are there threats associated with admission and treatment, but he must relate to new people too. If John is to manage that volume of change, then it is important for her to assess accurately how John is narrating the situation to himself. Care has to start with John's own perceptions. It would be inappropriate to simply load him with new information that he must quickly process. So relating starts well before hospital admission and with his existing carer. Later, John will be introduced to new carers, people with other expertise.

Here are three short excerpts of narrative that John shared with Alice. The first concerned the causation of cancer. John knew people sometimes did get cancer but he didn't have an accurate idea about why it happened.

When you eat the wrong things then that can make you ill. You mustn't put things in your mouth that are bad for you. I don't know what I ate that's bad, I don't know what I did wrong, but I don't want to do it again and I don't want the others to hate me because of it.

John's conception of the aetiology (the origin or cause) of cancer was limited. He knew that fibre was good for you (*eat your greens*), and that illness sometimes resulted from a *bad diet*. He knew that people sometimes suffered from tummy problems through eating germs. But he also seemed to identify a moral origin for the cancer, as though he was being punished for not eating properly. Alice was aware that some of John's reasoning templates centred quite strongly upon his now deceased mother, whom he missed. She had been very directive about his diet as they wrestled with weight control.

The second excerpt of narrative was associated with hospitals. Going to hospital could be necessary for quite small things: *people get their gall bladder out, Dorothy [John's friend] did.* But he was aware too that sometimes hospitals kept you there a long time, something that worried him greatly.

> *I suppose they decide how long they going to keep you once they got you. They decide and keep you till they ready to let you go. I don't know whether you can ask to go home, but maybe they say no.*

Alice noted the heavy emphasis on rules as John talked about hospital. John liked some rules, but those were rules that reassured. Rules that kept you away from friends might be bad rules. The residential community was a place of predictable order, and the hospital might not be; it would look, smell, sound and run differently.

John's third narrative concerned the *bag on your belly*. He had no clear idea of what this was or how it related to protecting the bowel while recovery from surgery proceeded. The cutting of bad bits out of you didn't seem entirely strange as you cut things out that weren't good to eat, but he didn't understand how he would pass poo onto his tummy and why he would need to change the bags attached so as to remain clean.

> *I don't know much about bags and your belly. What do you carry around at any road? What you put in that bag and why you have to carry it? I reckon that they cut a hole in you and they take out the bad bit. Then they sew you up. You don't need a bag.*

Activity 4.3   Critical thinking

What do you deduce from the short narrative excerpts shared above? They don't just focus on what the medical team think needs to be done. Do you think that matters?

An outline answer is given at the end of this chapter.

Practice tip

To help develop your ability to identify concerns and issues in a patient's narrative, arrange to take a patient history accompanied by a trusted colleague. After the interview both deliberate on what you thought chiefly concerned the patient and then compare notes. Hearing your colleague's interpretation will help you counter any tendency to interpret experience in a familiar way.

Alice's experience of working with John highlights the importance of working with his concerns first. Worries cannot simply be forced into cold storage. If they are not explored, then they may re-emerge later at difficult junctures in care. So even before she introduces Kieran, the liaison nurse who will help tell John about what is to come, she starts to tackle John's worries. Her willingness to listen attentively to what he explains is key to reassuring him about forthcoming care. If John's first concern (what causes bowel cancer) seems slightly abstract, it is nonetheless a priority matter for him. She gently corrects the notion that you catch bowel cancer from food and that it is possible to pass cancer on, for instance through a dining room. Yes, a lack of fibre in your diet (she exampled good things to eat) might make bowel cancer more likely, but you didn't catch cancer from food.

Activity 4.4 Critical thinking

Alice ensured that there was a private place to listen to John's worries and plenty of time to hear what he said. Her listening strategy was to invite him to explore his worries one at a time. It required a little judgement to decide when to ask him another question, something that helped her clarify exactly what he meant. If she interrupted too often, then he might falter in his narrative. If she let the account run, then there was a risk that it would be harder to return him to a point on which she was yet unclear of his concern. What do you think this tells us about the quality of listening that may be required in person-centred care?

An outline answer is given at the end of this chapter.

Alice next invited John to think about the length of a hospital stay. The doctors and nurses would want to check that John was recovered from his operation, but they wouldn't want to keep him a long time. The staff knew that he would miss his friends (notice the emphasis on personal needs) and that there would be other patients who might need an operation too. Hospital was a place where they planned things each day and checked that the patients were happy with that. The rules were arranged so that patients knew what would happen. There would, for example, be a rule about not eating just before the operation and then one about when he could start eating after it as well. This was to ensure that his gut had a chance to mend properly. Notice here how Alice selects examples of rules and their functions. She is eager to reassure John that the rules have a proper purpose. Notice too the emphasis upon a predictable ordering of the daily events. This was something that Alice knew John valued.

Alice explained that she had invited Kieran, a nurse from the hospital, to come and explain about the bag on his tummy and to describe what hospital was like. Kieran was going to be one of John's special nurses, someone who got to know him before he went to hospital.

There are some key points to take from this narrative analysis and Alice's response.

- Notice that the attention centres on John's concerns. Enough needs to be explained about cancer but we need to ensure that he is not overloaded with information. Soon, to support informed consent, however, the importance of the operation would need to be explained, but information is shared in manageable chunks.
- Alice is not afraid to correct a misapprehension, but it is done in such a way that John can see benefits too. There are some good foods to eat that help your gut remain healthy.
- Alice invited John to reason aloud about the length of his hospital stay. It can be tempting to reason for patients, to instruct and tell, but here Alice realises that John will feel more confident if he rehearses his own fears about a long hospital stay. The quick solution, that which addresses the medical problem, is often to instruct, but that doesn't necessarily address personal need.

Kieran (the liaison nurse) then visited to talk about the planned admission to hospital. Alice arranged for John to meet Kieran in the art studio (his favourite room) and for coffee to be available as they talked about what was planned in 10 days' time.

Activity 4.5   Reflection

What do you think the benefits of having Kieran come to meet John in his home are? Why is it valuable to have a liaison nurse such as Kieran? Once you've jotted an answer down, turn to my suggestions at the end of the chapter.

An outline answer is given at the end of this chapter.

Negotiating patient care (planning)

Alice and Kieran have shared a long telephone conversation before he comes to visit John in his home. They are keenly aware that they have to translate a medical problem into something that is personally comprehensible and tolerable for John. So whilst new information has to be shared, equal planning attention is given to anticipating the process of John's hospital stay. Table 4.1 contrasts the different requirements that Alice and Kieran have discussed when planning the meeting with John.

Table 4.1 Patient and hospital requirements

John's anticipated requirements To:	Hospital requirements To:
Move into a strange environment in which he would meet a range of new people.	Admit John on schedule and secure an adequately informed consent to surgery and any necessary post-operative treatment.
Establish a new daily routine, a way of adequately anticipating what would happen and why this would be beneficial.	Enable John to be nursed with a minimum of anxiety within a surgical ward.
Retain as far as was possible contact with trusted supporters.	Rehearse with him what would be different about his bowel function after surgery and how his abdomen would look. To teach him about an ostomy bag and its management until the bowel can be later re-anastomosed.
Ensure that he can communicate with a degree of confidence, others understanding and respecting what he said.	
Understand what the surgery would do and why an ostomy bag was needed.	Complete the operative preparations and safely anaesthetise him for surgery. Thereafter, assist him with a safe post-operative recovery.
Feel secure about going to sleep for the operation.	Manage his fluid and nutrient intake in a way that does not threaten planned surgery and which facilitates his bowel recovery afterwards.
Know where he was and what was happening when he recovered from surgery.	
Look after body function (going to the toilet) in a different way.	Assist him to manage his own stoma until he returns home.
	Help him anticipate a future operation to re-establish his normal bowel function (dependent on assessment of tumour resection, bowel health and stoma success).

Meeting John at the community home, Kieran explained to John that hospital was a place of new sensations, not only differently dressed staff, but strange smells and sounds as well. John's problems include features of autism spectrum disorder (Richards, 2017). John was hypersensitive to sensory stimuli; for example, strange noises worried him. Monitors or drip regulator alarms could create problems. It was important then to warn John that hospitals were sometimes noisy but that the noises were easily managed by the nurses. John had only to ask what they meant, and the nurses would explain.

Alice reminded John about Grace, who volunteered at the residential community but who also did hospital visits. Grace reminded John of his mother and she seemed a reassuring presence in his daily life. It might therefore be a good idea to see whether Grace could play a role as a companion for John during his hospital stay.

Agreeing a patient journey

Person-centred care work involves exploring the issues and challenges of what lies ahead and then modelling what might count as a solution (see Chapter 2). In the case of John, though, this requires that there is considerable emphasis on mapping future events in sequence. This is what will happen first, and then this. It is less appropriate to raise the problem starkly and then to offer the solution. Instead Kieran and Alice focus on telling a story of what lies ahead, embedding essential information (for informed consent and reassurance) along the way. Raising the prospect of Grace acting as a hospital companion for John then is not quite as 'cart before the horse' as we might imagine. Grace represents not a solution, but part of a continuity story about daily living in what is likely to seem a strange place.

Alice confirmed with Kieran that the hospital used a patient passport system (Northway et al., 2017). Kieran brought along a simple one-page passport that they used (see Figure 4.1). This included three boxes that he suggested they fill in with John before he came to hospital. The first box recorded things that John felt staff must understand about his needs and concerns. The second box related to what would help John as regards the style of communication used. For example, he might like explanations to be illustrated with a drawing. The third box related to what interested John about

Patient's Name: *John Beddows*   **Patient's ward:** *Onibury*
Ward extension number: *3714/3715*

My needs

I am having planned surgery on my bowel, but this sometimes seems complicated, so if you have investigations or treatments to explain I may need simple explanation and more time to understand what you say. The hospital seems big and strange, so it's possible I could get lost. It will help me if you guide me to where I need to go. Night time in a strange place makes me anxious, so remind me where I am.

Communication

I prefer to be called John. I can hear people fine, you don't need to shout, but please talk slowly and clearly. It will help me if you avoid any big medical words. Sometimes it helps if you explain something using a drawing. Thank you.

My stay

I like flowers and the gardens around the hospital. They make me feel calm. Feelings and complicated discussions I can't keep up with. My friend Grace is a special helper who comes with me around the hospital.

Figure 4.1 John's completed hospital passport

his hospital stay and what might enable him to feel curious about his care. Like other patients with a learning disability, Kieran wondered whether there were things that John might be fascinated by, eager to understand, as these could provide a greater sense of personal control.

The one-page passport was attached at the front of a patient's notes, but Kieran explained that he had also arranged for a summary to be produced in reduced A5 size that John could carry and show to any staff so that he didn't have to repeat his concerns. Alice was encouraged by that, as passport systems are only as good as the use made of them. That which remained filed was not that which assisted the patient (Drozd and Clinch, 2016).

Activity 4.6   Reflection

Pause now to consider how Alice and Kieran's opening negotiation of care with John seems to differ from how you have routinely acquainted surgical patients with what lies before them. To help you to do this, concentrate on the following:

a.   Do you routinely explain so much about the sequence of events and what each means?
b.   Do you routinely talk about requirements, problems and risks – that which care will counter – rather than story the hospital stay? (Problem and then solution versus events and reassurances.)
c.   Do you routinely help the patient anticipate the different healthcare professionals that they will meet and explain what they do?
d.   Do you notate with care what the patient specifically requests help with?

As this answer is based on your own reflection, there is no outline answer at the end of this chapter.

Practice tip

Not all patients can read or write, so jointly drafting a traditional written plan of care might be unrealistic. An alternative might be to audiotape the conversation about a planned hospital stay so that the shared narrative can be revisited to check that care remains what all parties anticipated.

Using research evidence

Alice explained to me that there was growing research about the combining of story-telling (ways in which patients anticipate events that will happen) with the use of a pre-operative visit to the hospital and the use of photographs (Blair et al., 2017). Patients were assisted if they were rehearsed in the sequence of events, hospital admission, pre-operative care, recovery and return to a ward, as this helped them to feel a sense of control. Simple, clear guides on going to hospital such as that by Hollins et al. (2015) were very useful, but Alice suggested that there was value in John preparing his own scrapbook about the forthcoming visit.

Some researchers (Gomez-Urquiza et al., 2016) have studied the benefit of using photographs to help patients with learning disabilities to manage their anxieties. In that study, patients chose pictures of nature and of their family to prompt distracting and reassuring thoughts, and that was combined with the use of favourite music recordings. The approach seemed to improve patient confidence and to aid recovery, when compared with simple reassurances offered by staff. Ginicola et al. (2015) had also observed the benefits of using photographs to support counselling work done with patients. Photographs could be used to help patients to focus on relevant issues and prompted a clearer articulation of their thoughts.

Kieran wondered how the different elements of preparatory care might fit together. It was routine to facilitate a pre-operative visit to the hospital for patients with special needs. That was augmented by staff members such as Alice talking over the sequence of planned events so that these were clear in the patient's mind. He asked, what if the photographs weren't taken from elsewhere? What if the staff were willing to have John take their photographs on his pre-admission visit, so that these could be printed off and added to his scrapbook? Might that not help too, enabling John to recognise quickly those people caring for him? Was it better to use photographs to distract and reassure the patient, or to brief and familiarise the patient with people he would meet?

Alice and Kieran asked John if he would like to visit the hospital in advance and to bring his camera so that he could take pictures of what he would see there. Kieran arranged for the ward sister, the anaesthetist and the surgeon to have their photographs taken too, so that these could be added to John's scrapbook. John said that he liked that idea if Grace could accompany him. It seemed of immense reassurance to him that he would have a friend visit regularly and that he could talk over what was happening with her.

Consent to surgery

Next, Kieran moved on to explore what John understood about his planned operation. While patients have varying capacity to understand complex concepts such as cancer and possible treatments, the Mental Capacity Act 2005 (Brown et al., 2015) makes it clear that every effort must be made to aid patients to make decisions in their own terms. So Kieran asked John to tell him why he thought the operation was being recommended. Here is an excerpt of John's response.

> *Well I have a cancer inside my guts and if they don't take it away it will get worse. They say that it could block me up or grow some place else in me. But if they cut it out, I should get better. It ain't going to stop me eating. I gotta eat the right things, but it ain't gonna stop me eating when I come home.*

Kieran asked John whether he thought it might be an uncomfortable operation.

They going to put me to sleep, so I don't feel it! Then, afterwards I can have tablets, my doctor said that. He said that they would get me up soon enough, I didn't have to stay in bed all the time. I could have tablets if I got sore.

Kieran felt reassured that John understood that surgery was important and that it could avert problems later on. He felt confident that John understood that he would be asleep whilst the operation was completed and would receive analgesia afterwards. We might debate whether a patient should be consulted on alternative treatments for cancer and apprised of the risks of disease recurrence, but in this instance, it seemed more appropriate to address the current problem, removing a circumscribed tumour and returning normal bowel function as promptly as possible.

What about the bag you will wear after the operation, what do you think that will be like?, Kieran wondered.

I'm going to have a bag on my tummy. But I can wear it under my shirt so people don't see, John answered.

Kieran wasn't sure how much John understood about that. He knew the sort of drawings that were used to show where on the body the bag was attached. But in his experience the illustrations weren't that satisfactory. They were always seen from the front and with nothing inside the bag. So, checking Alice's expression, he asked whether John might like to try a bag out. John agreed and so he unbuttoned his shirt and Kieran showed him the semi-opaque stoma bag that would be used. It had a hole in it through which the poo entered. Kieran showed how with his fingers.

Shall we make it the right weight, like it would be if you had some poo inside and you needed to change the bag? Kieran wondered. John agreed and Kieran pushed two pieces of a chocolate bar inside the bag. They laughed, but Kieran explained it was about the right weight. John could feel how it felt against his skin. Alice watched as the filled bag was attached.

Activity 4.7   Reflection

Jot down ideas now about the investment sometimes needed in the planning of care – that which seems necessary for a patient such as John. It happens well ahead of surgery. It may require an exploratory visit and focuses strongly on experiences and sensations. Notice Kieran's innovative way of helping John anticipate what it will feel like to wear an ostomy bag. Next, decide whether the care plan is always entirely contained within a written document. Whilst a written record is still required, what might be the limits of that if a patient has a learning disability?

An outline answer is given at the end of this chapter.

Collaborating in person-centred care (implementing)

Six days after his exploratory visit to hospital, the taking of many pictures of the building and its surrounding flower gardens, and meeting with key staff, John was admitted for his planned surgery. Grace and Alice accompanied him and a rota of visiting was agreed between the three of them and the ward sister, Loretta. Kieran visited John within an hour of his admission and together they reviewed how the scrapbook was filling up. John had collected pictures of the surgeon, anaesthetist, Kieran and the staff nurse, Willow, who specialised in ostomy care. Surgery was planned for the next day and it was arranged that Grace would be allowed to accompany John all the way into the anaesthetics room, where he would then go to sleep for his planned operation.

As part of his care package, staff on the ward were:

- acquainted with his hospital passport;
- asked to explain any sudden noises that might alarm John;
- advised to allow extra time when giving information prior to a clinical procedure (medical terminology should be avoided where possible);
- asked to rehearse with John the forthcoming events of the day so he could better understand the ward routine and any requests that might be made of him.

In Chapter 2 I detailed the sort of work associated with the collaborating stage of person-centred care, and I was eager to review with Kieran and Alice the extent to which such was possible with John. The surgery had been uneventful; a small section of his descending colon had been resected and sent to histology. A stoma was successfully formed on his abdominal wall and he was hydrated intravenously until his bowel sounds returned and small amounts of oral fluids were then begun. As arranged, Grace had remained on the hospital grounds and when John returned to the ward a little groggy, she was there to greet him and assure that all was well. Later that afternoon the surgeon visited him to tell him about what had been done. With the exception of saying that 'tissue had gone off for histology', the explanation was handled in very accessible layman's terms.

Collaborative work centres on clear roles and support. It centres on monitoring the comfort of the patient, alongside how they are progressing physically. It was important to monitor not only the post-operative patient (medical problem) but also the person who was coming to terms with what was likely to have been an anxiety-provoking passage of care. Kieran answered first.

> *I think we managed very well indeed; Loretta and I briefed all the ward staff about John's needs. We made a special point about how sudden noises could frighten him, we explained who Grace and Alice were and that we were offering extended visiting times for them.*

I described their work as helping John to narrate what had happened in the last hours and to reassure him about any matters that Loretta, Willow or I had not managed to explain.

Alice nodded and continued …

I was relieved too, the staff were very friendly. The woman who brought refreshments around seemed especially helpful and John looked forward to hearing her tell jokes about the weather. How one woman can know so many jokes about that I don't know! Anyway, we sat down each visit and asked John to bring us up to date on events. John seemed happy to proceed that way and then after the review we looked at his scrapbook.

I asked Alice how the scrapbook seemed to work as part of John's care.

He seemed to use it to open conversations with other people, she explained, rather than use it to distract himself from worries, he encouraged people to come and look through his photographs. He was especially pleased with the pictures of flowers that he had taken. He had made friends with Naomi, the tea lady, that way and one of the other patients had explained that he used to be a professional gardener.

Activity 4.8   Reflection

Alice imagined that the scrapbook would be used as a means of distracting John from his operation, worries about the stoma and subsequent self-care. She anticipated that it would help remind John of the world beyond the hospital walls. In fact, the scrapbook became a means of forming working relationships. Do you have any experience of care measures working differently to plan, but still beneficially? How important was it to think on your feet and repurpose care measures, so that they advance care?

An outline answer is given at the end of this chapter.

Both Kieran and Alice noted that John was noticeably relieved after the operation was completed and after he started to drink again. Prior to the surgery he had been polite but very quiet. He attended carefully to all that was explained to him but did not ask questions. After surgery, though, he seemed happier to converse and to explain his interests in gardening (not previously recognised by Alice and residential community staff). I wondered whether John spoke about his operation to the other patients or to Naomi, the tea lady. What seemed of particular interest in person-centred care terms was whether John was ready to relate an operation to others and beyond that, any remaining self-care challenges.

In person-centred care the patient's narrative is ongoing and it can take new directions at different times (Warmington, 2020). This is important and it justifies making care planning an incremental process. What seemed a good idea to begin with might need to be adjusted if the narrative subsequently changed. Patients might become frightened, more pessimistic; they might worry that progress cannot continue and, in the case of John, this seemed of particular concern. John had already shared his anxiety about staying in hospital longer than seemed strictly necessary.

Practice tip

It can be a good idea when reviewing an ongoing narrative with a patient to set the reflections in terms of what has just happened and what that means for next care. In this way you can monitor their grasp of cause-and-effect issues and the ways in which problems might be solved. Assessing what the patient anticipates imminently is a good way of assessing their discomfort and current coping.

Post-operative episodes

Kieran told me that they had identified three brief episodes during the post-operative days back on the ward and each had temporarily dented John's confidence. All of the episodes had occurred at a time when Grace and Alice were not present, so it was important for staff to produce holding solutions that would reassure John.

The first episode related to when John started to take oral fluids again. Willow had produced a stethoscope so that John could listen to his bowel sounds – that which signalled that he could slowly start to return to an oral diet. He then became distressed, though, because he said that once he started drinking again, the hole in his tummy would leak everywhere. He was reluctant to drink because the stoma was for poo and if his drink came out too, then he would wet the bed and make a mess.

Activity 4.9   Reflection

Pause for a moment to consider how much you think the patients that you have nursed understand their own physiology. Did that matter with regard to what you explained about an operation? Patients vary in the degree to which they need to master information about body function (see Chapter 5), but with a patient who lives with a learning disability, there may arise surprises because of what they do not know. Person-centred care focuses strongly upon experiences and emotions linked to that. If an experience seems likely to be threatening, then it is often necessary to rehearse why it happens.

As this answer is based on your own reflection, no outline answer is given at the end of the chapter.

Kieran realised that in explaining the operation to John and how the bag would help, he had focused entirely on solids. However helpful the ostomy bag demonstration was, it had not helped John anticipate what might happen when he drank fluids. At this stage, John had not looked at his stoma but he realised that the covering dressing had once seemed very damp. Now the nurse had to assure John that drinking was safe and indeed important. She had to explain that the bowel absorbed a great deal of fluid before it reached John's stoma.

The second critical episode had occurred during night shift. John had received post-operative analgesia but then woke in the dark, feeling the need to urinate. At this stage he had already begun mobilising, walking with assistance to the ward toilet. In the dark, however, the geography of the ward seemed entirely different. John pressed his call bell, requesting assistance, but when none arrived quickly he shuffled to the toilet himself. Having completed that, he then took a wrong turn in the dark and proceeded into another bay where female patients were being nursed. One woman raised the alarm when she saw John standing confused at the foot of her bed and John had been gently led back in the right direction. The next morning John was subdued, feeling that he had transgressed the rules of the ward. He worried that they might not let him go home because he got lost.

Kieran took time to explain that a strong post-operative analgesia can sometimes 'muddle thought' and that in the dark, a strange place was confusing for everyone. He had simply got lost and the other patient was entirely reassured that he had meant no harm. What determined his discharge ('going home time') from hospital was solely an assessment of when he was ready to do so, looking after himself back in the residential community.

The third episode related to the feel of his stoma. Willow had warned him that it would look 'pink and shiny' but she had not warned him that it would not feel the same as his skin. When he gently touched his stoma, learning to clean it, the sensations were not at all the same. Yet because it looked red and sore, he imagined that it would be very sensitive to his touch. At first this seemed a relief to John, but then the nurse encouraged him to walk straight rather than bowed forward. He resisted the request and it was only later that Loretta learned that John feared that to stretch upright might be to break his gut and have to stay in hospital. *It might snap*, he said, *then they will have to operate again and pull it out.* Loretta encouraged him to straighten gently and to watch his exposed stoma when he did that. It remained firmly in place.

The three critical incidents are instructive about this stage in person-centred care:

- they highlight just how powerful perceptions are in shaping patient behaviour and responses to care suggestions. John's perceptions are largely misguided, but it is quite possible for patients to harbour perceptions, to form beliefs, that might limit or even derail care;

- they raise the question of whether it is possible to entirely insulate a patient from problems. In John's case extensive work was done to model what care would look and feel like. However, John, as other patients, encountered unanticipated problems and then reassurance needed to be as clear and simple as possible;

- it is usually necessary to return to the patient's perceptions in order to ensure that they feel able to liaise with you on care measures. It would have been easy for the night staff nurse to simply report that John had got lost in the dark, but that might then have been to misunderstand his more withdrawn demeanour the following day. John connected the confusion at night to rule breaking and he needed reassurance about that.

John made excellent progress learning to manage his own stoma bag. Willow showed him how the bags were scented to help hide the smell of his poo. She took pictures on his camera for him with and without the bag, hidden beneath his shirt. John asked Alice if she could tell the difference between the two photographs and she could not. Because the stoma was not sore and his skin remained very sound, John found it easy to attach the bag to his skin. He began to mobilise confidently and to enjoy a series of small meals as he checked the effect that this had on his stoma. Willow showed him the foods that made it more likely that he would produce a better-formed stool, that which was then easier to manage. Then the surgeon came to tell John that there was no evidence that the cancer had spread beyond the piece of gut he had removed, and that he could go home again. His health would be monitored in the coming months but it would be a good idea to then come and have his gut repaired so that he did not need to use a bag anymore. John was delighted.

Evaluating person-centred care (evaluating)

John's personal evaluation of the hospital stay was one of relief. He didn't like the smell of the place, that it was so busy, but he had liked Naomi, the tea lady, and now he wondered if he could help the gardener who managed the grounds at the residential community. The operation had made him a little sore and he didn't like that he couldn't (for now) go to the toilet his usual way, but he understood that one more operation would help return that to normal. Alice asked John about how Kieran, Willow and Loretta had seemed and he affirmed that they were very nice indeed. Alice pressed him, *nice in what way?*, but John insisted that they were just nice. You were nice or not nice. There weren't variants of nice.

Anticipating a return hospital visit in the future, Kieran rang Alice to review how the care support had gone from her and Grace's perspective. They reviewed it using the PERSON mnemonic that they had chosen at the start of the episode.

Perception

Kieran and Alice agreed that they had a reasonably good understanding of John's perceptions: the fear of being delayed in hospital and the concerns about how cancer began in his bowel. Grace had added useful observations from what John told her. But there was, Kieran acknowledged, a weakness regarding how he conceived of bowel function and hydration. A little more explanation was needed about what a stoma was, an opening of the bowel itself onto the abdomen. Willow had had to tidy up that explanation. The importance of noise as a possible threat for John had been remembered late on and countered with staff briefing.

Explore

Alice said that she had prior knowledge about John's life and so she had possibly been a little complacent, assuming some things that he would need. For example, the scrapbook had been conceived as a distractor from current worries and John had used it in quite another way. Alice was surprised that she had not realised John's interest in gardening, but that was now something she and he could build upon.

Relate

Both colleagues felt pleased with the efforts made to relate warmly and supportively to John. Loretta, Willow, Naomi, the surgeon and the anaesthetist had all adjusted their approach to acknowledge John's needs. Grace, the volunteer, in particular, had proven an anchor for John as he was admitted and then prepared for surgery. What was less clear was whether spur-of-the-moment nurse responses to John's expressed concerns were as refined as they might have been. Kieran observed that colleagues sometimes forgot about the need to explain slowly and then to check again that a patient such as John was happy to proceed. The hospital passport had been used comparatively rarely and may have functioned as a token reassurance for John.

Source

Alice concluded that both she and Kieran had worked well to explore John's fears and needs. The investment in narrative analysis was considerable but it had probably contributed to John's positive attitude towards the follow-up operation. If John was not expressive about his hospital stay, then he did not express dismay either. Kieran and colleagues would have a reasonable base to start from at his next hospital admission.

Outline

Centring the care planning on a journey, explaining what would happen each day, had been a success. Loretta had set this down in the care plan record, but it wasn't something that was easy to express in goals and action terms. The point was that a plan required considerable flexibility as staff monitored John's narrative each day. Something more mechanistic would not capture that. Nonetheless, the goal of rehearsing with John the planned daily events had worked well, and John clearly valued what he thought of as his 'look-ahead' chat.

Notify

Alice and Kieran were satisfied with the care liaison measures – the ways in which other staff had been briefed and engaged in John's care. What remained to be seen was whether they would develop best working principles to help other patients with a learning disability. John's care had consisted of more than the standard pre-surgery hospital visit. The investment seemed to avert any major crises, and it represented a good investment of hospital resources.

Case study insights

I would suggest that there are four major insights to take away from John's case study.

Investing time and expertise

The first is that some care requires a significant investment of time and expertise. For John to transition to the hospital experience in a way that prepared him for a later return and possibly other cancer treatment required a great deal of frontloaded work on the part of Alice, Kieran and Grace, the volunteer. Reviewed in cost–benefit terms, the investment seems worthwhile, not only in terms of dignity and security for John, but also in terms of a relatively smooth package of hospital care. A frightened and agitated patient could threaten the ward environment and perhaps even treatment itself. None of that investment, though, makes sense unless narrative analysis forms the basis for care planning.

Strategic liaison work

The second insight is that sometimes person-centred care relies heavily upon strategic liaison work. Remove Kieran or Alice from the care episode, their expertise, and it seems unlikely that John would have had such a successful hospital stay. In circumstances such as these it seems unlikely that any one individual will have all the knowledge and skills to negotiate care in a way that adequately suits a patient such as John. There are likely to be many care episodes that are less polished and as attentive as this one, but which remain nonetheless something that care staff can build upon.

Creating a care environment

The third insight is that much of the work completed here was to create and sustain a supportive care environment. The surgery, pre-operative checks and post-operative physical care measures remain as before, but what is attended to differently is the communication shared with John. Creating a supportive care environment can be seen as a capital investment if staff positively evaluate the care delivered and anticipate with pride the ability to repeat similar useful measures to suit another patient. As was suggested in Part 1 of this book, person-centred nursing care is deeply psychological. How we listen, what we say and what we do operates in the realm of perceptions and feelings and it can help build a relationship of trust.

Working with personal narratives

The fourth insight is that narrative analysis is important to the delivery of successful person-centred care. Looking back over the case study, you might have remarked just how much attention Alice in particular gives to listening to John's narrative of concerns and experiences. The work began the moment that John was investigated for bowel cancer and tests were completed. But it grew apace and in intensity once the diagnosis of cancer was made and a best-treatment course of action was proposed to John. I wonder how that made you feel. Could you explore a patient narrative in the same way? What would it entail to explore perceptions in this manner?

It's fair to observe that Alice is highly experienced in understanding the needs of service users with a learning disability. She is attuned to the way they talk about themselves and the world about them. When I asked her about that, whether it was a knack or a skill, about what it took to explore a narrative in such depth, she couldn't initially explain how she proceeded. It had become intuitive to her and she barely paused to plan the next question, to set the next scene that would enable someone to explore their thoughts aloud. Two days later, though, she came back to me with an email examining what was involved in exploring a personal narrative in such an intensive way.

She explained that it was important to start with modest expectations and to assure oneself that what was revealed might not immediately be understandable or resolvable. Working in the residential community setting, there was ample time for narratives to be revisited. There was scope to observe residents, the better to appreciate what they were feeling or saying. Body language, social interactions, all built on the information that might be gleaned in a private discussion. She appreciated that nurses working in other settings, especially acute care, did not have the luxury of such long periods of observation and reflection. Responses to narratives had to be quicker and quite probably not so finely tuned. Nonetheless, deciding in advance that your enquiry had to be perfect was the wrong way to begin. Even modest beginnings were helpful.

Alice remembered that her first ever worries about encouraging service users to narrate their experiences centred on what they might then expect of her, the nurse. *If I ask, then I save*, she said, recounting that this eventually seemed an impossible promise. As counsellors realise, the emotional, psychological work of coping remains in large part that of the patient. To enquire about experiences, feelings and thoughts was to facilitate whatever level of coping the patient could muster. That was even true for someone such as John. In exploring his narrative she and Kieran had worked to set out support provision in hospital that made coping easier. But much of the rehearsal of thoughts too was designed to help John reassure himself about what would happen and how he would then be able to cope. So Alice's first advice was: don't hold back from enquiring because you believe that you must be *the complete solution*. What you discover was always there, but perhaps unconsidered. If there is a problem, then it is better to realise that in a calm environment rather than have it possibly erupt unexpectedly later on.

In her email to me she emphasised that even after John's hospital stay she was still discovering new things about how he thought and felt. So it was important to be patient with yourself as well. You will not understand everything that you hear immediately. A narrative analysis conversation is not a definitive, never-changing insight into another human being. It is simply the beginning of discovery and it offers up puzzles. Whilst she knew that John thought in a very rule-bound way, it wasn't immediately clear where or how he linked ideas about illness, eating and being good together. The question was, though, whether narrative exploration was worth embarking upon for the hospital stay planned.

Alice said, listening intently to John was not just about understanding his fears and needs, it was about telling him that they mattered. I don't entirely know how much of a difference that made to him. This is a man who doesn't spell out things so clearly.

People are nice or not nice. So it's difficult to judge how much listening and then planning mattered to him. Nonetheless, it seems to me likely that they did matter. When I asked Alice to review how often John became distressed at home, she confirmed that this might happen once or perhaps twice a week. If he faced sudden change, if situations seemed especially ambiguous to him, then he could easily become verbally aggressive. It seemed, then, entirely possible that for John to spend time in hospital and to return home, managing his stoma, without such an episode was a significant achievement.

Just what else did enquiring into a narrative entail, then? Well, it required judgement. *You feel an urge to clarify what someone like John says every few moments*, she explained, and this was because you want to arrange care that fits as well as possible. But it was important to realise that the urge to ask so many clarification questions, about what John meant, was often for her own benefit. Some questions were asked because she doubted her ability to interpret what he said. People with a learning disability sometimes reasoned in peculiar ways. She had learned over time, though, that if you managed to persuade someone to think aloud, they would sometimes run a narrative for several minutes at a time as they discovered their feelings about an issue. If you were patient, then the answers to your queries might pop out of the continuing narrative. If you could but master your urgent need to understand what the service user said, you might both assure the individual that you listened well and secure the more complete, rounded account of their thoughts.

Alice had one final point to make in her email. She explained that inviting someone to narrate their feelings and concerns sometimes meant that you secured after-thought information. John, and others sometimes, returned to a thought that was bothering them, perhaps hours later. It was a good idea therefore to be ready to note down what they subsequently offered. You might wonder whether it was then necessary to return intently to another perhaps lengthy conversation. Alice's experience, though, was that this was rarely necessary. Most after-thought information seemed to fulfil a tidying-up function. It might be to reassure the nurse that what was discussed had been thought about responsibly. Alice said,

> *Residents sometimes tell me extra things, little afterthoughts, and often that seems to serve an 'I'm alright and thank you for asking' function. John once said to me, 'you never seem to get upset'. I think that it surprised him when he often did. It was as if he felt that we were sponges, soaking up his excess anxiety.*

Narrative analysis and care strategy

After finishing my correspondence with Alice I paused to ponder exactly how her narrative analysis work had been used to serve a person-centred care strategy. Manifestly the narrative discussions with John were not formally counselling. Whilst they might serve to help enhance his confidence that he might cope with the operation and hospital stay, they were not therapeutic in the sense that we might understand it, for instance, with regard to psycho-analysis. Nor did Alice prescribe for John a series of cognitive behavioural techniques designed to help him reason through change on a day-to-day basis. The nearest care got to such therapy was the use of a scrapbook that Alice imagined might be used to distract John from anxious thoughts, but which was used instead to broker friendships with hospital staff and other patients. This seems important, for if you imagine that narrative analysis automatically equates to counselling, I think that you would be wrong. Whilst a form of cognitive behavioural work was used with Abraham in Chapter 3, narrative analysis did not here automatically result in a formal kind of therapy. In day-to-day social life people act as friends, enabling others to rehearse aloud their concerns. No pretence is made that solutions will necessarily be recommended, nor does the friend pretend to be a therapeutic authority. In a very tangible sense, Alice and others acted as friends to John, helping to carry him through a difficult period. Grace in particular functioned as a go-to person who would always take an interest in John's concerns during her hospital visits.

So what was narrative analysis used for on this occasion? I wonder if you agree that it was to anticipate the possible extent of John's coping within a new and more challenging circumstance. By listening to John's narrative, Alice was able to assess the nature of the cancer threat as John understood it. She and Kieran were able to understand John's command of information relating to surgery and the subsequent ostomy bag. In listening to him they were able to observe his body language, the pitch of his voice, clues that would signal the extent of his distress. Arriving at an idea of what he found threatening and assessing whether that distressed him, they were able to formulate a better idea of needs. That pattern of needs was very individual. Few of us, for instance, would remark particularly upon noises in a hospital. Few might worry about a length of hospital stay if such was linked to obvious clinical need.

Once Alice and Kieran had a better understanding of John's likely needs, they were able to turn their attention to adjustments that might be possible within the care environment. That focused, for instance, on the benefits of a hospital visit, the scrapbook and use of photographs; it centred less successfully on the use of a hospital passport. The strategy centred on modifying the care environment to keep it as close as possible to John's coping ability. They manipulated the environment to match a little more closely John's needs. Whilst this still represented a major investment of time and effort, I would suggest that the cost was widely shared. The medical staff were asked to think for a moment about how they described the operation. Kieran used his imagination to make using an ostomy bag seem that much more real and yet achievable. So in many ways the strategy was to invest early to secure benefits for John, but it was also to ask a wider range of staff to adjust their care approach in relatively small ways. I wonder if you think, like me, that this was remarkably good. It wasn't a vastly new provision; it didn't require the import of expensive new talent. It consisted of joining up ideas to make personal care that much more plausible.

Chapter summary

Many idealistic conceptions of person-centred care are based upon partnership equality: patient and nurse offering equal but quite different contributions towards care. The case study of John, however, exemplifies what can still be achieved when one of the partners in care starts with a significant disadvantage. It demonstrates what can be done where a nurse or other primary care professional acts as the service user's advocate. Quintessentially, this very threatening medical problem (bowel cancer) was countered through insights into the personal needs of the patient. The personal problem (dealing with a hospital stay as well as surgery) took precedence and medical treatment was facilitated because of the way that nurses and others understood and supported the patient.

Activities: Brief outline answers

Activity 4.1 Reflection (p75)

I think that the most compelling advantage of this mnemonic is that it encourages the nurse to enquire and to listen to the patient. So much within hospital care focuses on the medical problem rather than the personal problem or need and PERSON helps to counterbalance that. Whilst you may have reservations about your own ability to analyse patient perceptions, to interpret a narrative shared, I believe that this mnemonic and the case study of John should help you to make a start. John lives in a world dominated by perceptions because he has rather less scope to reason beyond. It is then vital that we explore his understanding of the world around him.

Activity 4.2 Critical thinking (p77)

Even as a practised academic, a conference paper still seems a challenge to me, but it might have seemed a little more daunting to you. To do something new, in a new environment, with such a big audience seems to turn a spotlight on 'performance'. Am I good enough to do this, can I convince the audience that I have something to offer? When faced with such challenges we might try to remember past performances, perhaps a poetry recital at school, or offerings in a school debate. We also perhaps remember how past teachers structured a lecture. We imagine what might help the audience, remembering features of lectures that helped us. The extent to which we can do this depends on the ability to conceptualise the challenge, for example breaking it down into subjects to be taught, the best sequence in which to explain things and the time available. For John and others that might seem impossible.

Did you notice, though, how John has started to story bowel cancer at the end of the passage? He perhaps sees it as something which infects him, or perhaps something that happens when you are in a state of disgrace. He is feeling his way to an explanation, even if it is an inaccurate one and excludes him from social contact at mealtime.

Activity 4.3 Critical thinking (p78)

I wonder if the narratives seem irrational to you, highlighting something unusual about how John thinks. He worries about issues and experiences in a different way to you. He picks up ideas, template explanations, and extends them further, beyond that which evidence could support. His last narrative is one of ignorance, perhaps denial, but it is still important. It might be tempting to dismiss John's concerns as not important because they don't centre on the *real* problem ahead. But if you did, then that would be a mistake, for a patient behaves towards you not on the basis of logic or science. He may weave your attitudes, behaviour or words into a misguided explanation of events. It is in such circumstances then that conflict can arise.

Activity 4.4 Critical thinking (p79)

Alice needs to listen very hard; she has to attend to John's words with care. She dares not assume what he means. To listen is to do more than simply to hear; we have to interpret what is being said and that raises of the question of if and when we interrupt to clarify things. Nurses working in mental healthcare and support of people with learning disabilities become expert in this, but all nurses need the skill to practise well.

Activity 4.5 Reflection (p80)

I believe that John will feel more comfortable discussing change on 'home territory' and with the close support of someone that he trusts. The bridge to a strange place (hospital) starts in a safe place. John might reason that Kieran could be sent away; that he could readily refuse to go to hospital from such a vantage position. Kieran as a liaison nurse reduces the stress of transiting from safety to a strange place. He becomes a familiar face in a hospital full of new faces.

Activity 4.7 Reflection (p85)

We can think of John's psychological care as frontloaded and designed to create a safer environment in his mind. The reward is likely to be a less anxious patient and perhaps a more cooperative one too. In a busy hospital environment, both of these things are important. Nurses have to meet the needs of different patients, with finite resources, so if problems and needs can be anticipated beforehand, then so much the better. It is possible to outline requirements on a care plan, for instance as regards communication approach, information sharing and giving consent, but much of the care in such patient circumstances resides in the style of approach, the manner of care delivery, and that is often briefed and reiterated in ward handover reports. John's care follows precepts, but it responds daily to a changing narrative as well.

Activity 4.8 Reflection (p87)

Sometimes care benefits from discoveries along the way; it is iterative. This may be especially common in person-centred care where measures are negotiated and rely so strongly on communicated narratives. In a busy surgical ward that might sound overly complex, perhaps too fussy, but the point is that medical problems are only addressed if we attend to personal ones as well. Imagine a patient who fails to learn stoma self-care or whose stoma site breaks down with an infection because they don't follow self-care guidance. Such a patient may spend an extended time in hospital with the costs and challenges this entails. Working flexibly with personal needs can become a very good investment.

Further reading

One of the risks associated with nurse education is that we succumb to silo reading. What I mean by that is that we only read textbooks and articles relating to our own field of nurse education. The story of John above, though, demonstrates how short-sighted such a policy would be. Kieran needed to understand things about learning disability and Alice needed to understand the essentials of cancer treatments and stoma care. The following books will help you reach beyond some traditional boundaries, through study of personal narratives and what this means for healthcare.

Glintborg, C and de la Mata, M (eds) (2021) *Identity Construction and Illness: Narratives in Persons with Disabilities.* London: Routledge.

The editors introduce you to range of case study individuals who vividly convey their stories of illness, confusion, misunderstanding and what sometimes impresses as a rescue. Whilst you might only encounter some such patients in your professional work, what reading case studies offer you are glimpses of how people might think. This can help inoculate you against doubt and encourage you to enquire with patients, for nothing is entirely surprising if you have already read about the possibilities of experience.

Moore, D, Murphy, E and Nicholson, R (2019) *Bodies of Truth: Personal Narratives on Illness, Disability, and Medicine.* Lincoln, NE: University of Nebraska Press.

This is another collection of case study narratives, but possibly a more literary take on the subject. When you finish this book you may think, goodness, I never thought about healthcare like that! I never actually thought that patients might see us, as well as their problems, in this way! In this regard the book feels liberating; healthcare can be and do different things. But remember, first things first: if you are learning the basic skills, then they have to be mastered now and only later should you explore different conceptions of treatment or care.

Osgood, T (2020) *Supporting Positive Behaviour in Intellectual Disabilities and Autism: Practical Strategies for Addressing Challenging Behaviour.* London: Jessica Kingsley Publishers.

I confess to a dislike for very long titles in healthcare textbooks, but if that irritates you as well, set it aside and take a look at Osgood's selection of challenges in intellectual disability and account of how healthcare systems sometimes contribute to the problems. In my experience many nurses working in acute healthcare have only a limited insight into what is required to support people with a learning disability well. Much, for instance, relating to autism has been established in relatively recent times. So if you are not studying in this field of nurse education, this book represents a valuable read. If you are studying there, then you may yet discover new issues and debates through a better understanding of narratives and discourses that exist there.

Useful websites

Dang, B, Westbrook, R, Njue, S and Giordano, T (2017) Building trust and rapport early in the new doctor–patient relationship: a longitudinal qualitative study. *BMC Medical Education, 17* (32). https://doi.org/10.1186/s12909-017-0868-5

This is an open-access journal article that I would encourage you to read, the better to understand rapport and how patients sometimes see healthcare professionals. It concerns research with HIV-positive patients, in some regards a very different group to those who seek care and have a learning disability. But what I hope you will take away from it is how several patient concerns are probably widespread and recurring. Anxiety about illness and treatment is commonplace. Patients assume that we are knowledgeable, but what they hope to discover is that we have regard for their experience of a health problem.

The Challenging Behaviour Foundation: **www.challengingbehaviour.org.uk**

Not all patients with a learning disability exhibit challenging behaviour; that which can alarm healthcare staff, family carers and the wider public. John, for instance, became agitated relatively infrequently and then he was verbally rather than physically aggressive. Challenging behaviour may be more common where individuals are profoundly disabled and struggle emotionally to understand what is happening to them. The problem is, though, that nurses might fear that almost any patient can suddenly become aggressive. They may worry about exploring narratives in case distress and anger is suddenly triggered. This website offers further insight into challenging behaviour through a series of fact sheets. The site as a whole is worth exploring, the better to understand family as well as service user needs.

Chapter 5

Case study three

Helping Tom learn about diabetes

NMC Future Nurse Standards of Proficiency for Registered Nurses

This chapter will address the following platforms and proficiencies:

Platform 1: Being an accountable professional

At the point of registration, the registered nurse will be able to:

1.9 understand the need to base all decisions regarding care and interventions on people's needs and preferences, recognising and addressing any personal and external factors that may unduly influence your decisions.

Platform 2: Promoting health and preventing ill health

At the point of registration, the registered nurse will be able to:

2.10 provide information in accessible ways to help people understand and make decisions about their health, life choices, illness and care.

Platform 3: Assessing needs and planning care

At the point of registration, the registered nurse will be able to:

3.4 understand and apply a person-centred approach to nursing care, demonstrating shared assessment, planning, decision making and goal setting when working with people, their families, communities and populations of all ages.

Platform 4: Providing and evaluating care

At the point of registration, the registered nurse will be able to:

4.2 work in partnership with people to encourage shared decision-making, in order to support individuals, their families and carers to manage their own care when appropriate.

Introduction

In this third of the case studies, we turn to a young man (Tom) who is learning to manage diabetes mellitus. Whilst the case study covers each of the different stages of the person-centred care relationship, particular focus falls upon the planning and implementation of a teaching plan (negotiating and collaborating stages of person-centred care). In a wide variety of chronic illness contexts person-centred care will require the nurse to teach and the patient to learn. The imperatives of the medical problem (e.g. managing metabolic imbalances in diabetes) demand that the patient learn about their illness and ways to manage that. The personal problem is to accommodate the necessary life changes required and to learn in ways that seem both safe and motivating. The goal of patient education is then to protect and to facilitate a lifestyle that is both adaptive and meaningful during a stressful time.

Teaching patients

Learning to teach is an increasingly important part of the nursing curriculum. It is important with regard to correcting or managing illness, but sustaining wellness and public health as well (Miller and Stoeckel, 2017). There are too few clinicians to manage every chronic illness personally, so it is necessary for patients and lay carers to learn self-care. Not only will successful learning enable nurses to reserve sufficient support for patients who are acutely ill, but it will enable chronically ill patients to develop a greater self-esteem as they overcome the challenges posed by illness.

While you may have quite clear ideas about the teaching relationship in other settings, such as college, the relationship in healthcare is different (Price, 2015). For one thing, the learner may find themselves in the learning role quite suddenly. It can be difficult to begin learning if illness seems overwhelming. For another, the nurse, unlike the college teacher, does not have the same powers to assess and judge the performance of the learner. The nurse's 'student' is also a consumer, and the teaching on offer represents a part of service that the patient judges. While the teaching agenda may relate to the known challenges of a disease or treatment regimen (medical problem), the patient's perceived learning needs may more frequently be linked to what the patient has felt or worried about (personal problem) (Laursen et al., 2017a). What is then done first, what is emphasised and how things are taught have to address both of the problems before us.

Teaching patients about their illness and its management can be conceived of in different ways (see Table 5.1). You may have already been engaged in some elements of teaching even though the work was not labelled as such. However, in this chapter I conceive of teaching as something that is strategic, designed and arranged using techniques that help the patient increase their independence. Teaching here centres on facilitating the patient's learning, enabling them to identify goals of their own, and negotiating learning work in a sequence that helps to both reassure and motivate them. Facilitated learning is the educational equivalent of person-centred care (Price, 2015). We begin with the patient's perceptions – their understanding of risks and needs – and build on that with learning activities that seem sustaining to them. Teaching is certainly a form of psychological support; it is helpful, but it remains honest as well. If the patient fails to partner the nurse in the learning journey, then they may face multiple consequences, poorer health and additional problems in the future.

Table 5.1   Elements of teaching

Teaching element	Limitations and strengths
Informing	If we tell a patient about their illness, a drug or other treatment, then we have not yet taught them. We have simply given them information, much as patient leaflets and guidance sheets do (Sustersic et al., 2017). We cannot guarantee that they have learned anything, nor have we necessarily arranged the information in the way that makes the clearest sense to the patient. Nevertheless, informing has a role to play in patient education. Were we to ask the patient to find out things for themselves, they might secure guidance that is less evidence-based. We must therefore inform patients.
Explaining and guiding	Teaching involves explanation and guidance; we need to match this to the medical problem (what the patient needs to learn for safety and progress) and to the patient problem (finding best ways to regain control of their health). Nurses explain and guide a great deal, but if this is arranged in a haphazard way, then the patient might become confused and demoralised. So we need to explain and guide as part of an agreed strategy.
Demonstrating/ instructing	Nurses demonstrate things like injections, dressing techniques and catheter or stoma management. As the patient then tries techniques for themselves, we might instruct them, gently correcting their technique so that it is safe, more comfortable and effective (e.g. Anuradha, 2015). It would be unwise, however, to assume that once demonstrated, a skill is mastered. We need to check how confident the patient feels, to watch and reassure them as they try out the technique themselves.

Teaching element	Limitations and strengths
Supporting/ counselling	Learning involves emotional work – overcoming doubt, for example (Jones et al., 2019). It is by no means certain that patients immediately believe that they can manage an illness. So we need to teach in ways that build confidence. Counselling in this context is usually low key; we suggest ways to conceive of problems and to find solutions. If we help the patient master self-care, then we may free them from recurring problems for years ahead.
Checking and monitoring	Patients learning sometimes falter, so we will need to monitor and check their progress (e.g. Levy et al., 2018). It may be necessary to refer them to other teachers or support groups. This requires a readiness to watch their self-care work and to gently intervene, to correct or to advise. Such intervention isn't easy, however, as patients struggle for self-control. They can readily feel chastised by someone who seems to 'always know best'.
Assessing	We don't make patients sit examinations, but we do need to reassure them when we believe that they have mastered the necessary skills (Bastable, 2017). So here assessment fulfils a reward function (well done!) as well as judgement function (e.g. 'we need to go over the drug dosage calculation again, don't we, for your safety'). This work can seem strange to nurses who think of themselves as supporters and helpers rather than examiners.

Practice tip

Whilst watching a more experienced nurse teach a patient, concentrate hard on how the patient reacts and responds. How does teaching seem to register with the patient? All teachers need to remain acutely aware of learner reactions.

Activity 5.1   Reflection

Think back now to work that you have done with a patient who suffered from a chronic illness and who needed to adjust their life as a result. Did you practise any of the elements of teaching outlined in Table 5.1? Was that work done as part of a planned strategy? Did you, for instance, explore what learning goals the patient had? Was your work modified by the patient's own assessment of need?

As this answer is based on your own reflection, there is no outline answer at the end of the chapter.

The elements of teaching briefly outlined above are often linked to different stages of the patient's illness and to their learning preferences and aptitudes (see Table 5.2). Sharing information and explaining an illness and first treatment is often associated with acute illness circumstances. While this perhaps seems a less person-centred activity, it can fit well with the patient's circumstances. When the patient is acutely ill, the capacity to learn a great deal is limited. Patients typically suffer from information overload while at the same time dealing with strange new environments (Avery et al., 2016).

Table 5.2   Conceptions of teaching, stages of illness and patient ability assumptions

Stage of illness	Conception of teaching	Patient ability assumptions
Acute illness (something discovered and to be made sense of).	Sharing key information, informing the patient about the illness and principal treatment. The illness is stabilised.	The patient can understand the information provided and appreciates what additional questions to ask.
Recovering from illness and preliminary rehabilitation.	Teaching as demonstration, explanation and question-answering (making sense of circumstances). Work centres on helping patients to gain a first sense of control.	The patient is motivated to enquire and is attentive to what is shared by the nurse.
Dealing with a chronic illness, that which the person must self-manage to a significant degree.	Teaching now draws on a range of elements to suit patient needs. The patient is challenged to partner the nurse more and to anticipate future challenges that their learning can help them counter.	The patient is a proactive, inquisitive and highly motivated individual who seeks to regain and retain as much control over an illness-mediated life as possible.

Activity 5.2   Critical thinking

Table 5.2 raises an implicit teaching challenge, determining whether or not the patient is ready to learn. Medical pressures, for instance on available beds, might press care measures ever onwards, leaving less time to teach. What other questions do you think you might have to answer about the patient before you can begin to help educate them?

An outline answer is given at the end of this chapter.

Whilst teaching strategies will vary with patient circumstance and resources available to the nurse, three principles can usefully guide the educational work (Price, 2015):

1. First, counter what seems the greatest risk, that which could harm the patient. We have to stabilise the patient before they can become receptive learners; they need to feel safe first of all.

2. Second, understand what concerns the patient most of all and work upon those perceptions. Attending to patient worries promptly helps build rapport and increases the trust that will be needed to help them explore what is required to manage their illness.

3. Having secured first progress on the above, move towards that which expands the patient's understanding and sense of control and which will help them to reduce the risk of problems later on. Moving in this stepwise approach reassures the patient that they can learn incrementally, increasing their control as they proceed.

Case study: Tom

Tom is 14. He has recently suffered from a winter chest infection that proved extremely difficult to overcome and he spent a period of several months feeling exhausted. He had suffered from some skin infections too and had problems concentrating on his lessons. While being investigated for these problems, Tom's blood glucose levels were assessed and it was confirmed that he suffered from Type 1 diabetes mellitus. Tom has spent a short time in hospital where his blood glucose was regulated using intravenous infusions and he commenced insulin injections subcutaneously. A nurse on the ward demonstrated to Tom how he should check his blood sugar levels and then draw up the right insulin to inject himself with. The demonstration steps approach used are summarised in Table 5.3. Tom and his mother Naomi have been given information leaflets about Type 1 diabetes mellitus and they watched a short video on the altered physiology of the condition, but now they visit the diabetes clinic of the hospital and meet Chloe, the diabetes specialist nurse.

Tom seems nervous in the clinic. In truth, the news that he has diabetes stunned him. He thought that old people got that condition. His mother, in sharp contrast, seems relieved. She admits that she feared Tom might have had cancer when he started to lose weight. For Naomi now, care is all about getting down to the business of controlling what you eat and how you self-administer insulin. She has watched the nurse inject Tom with insulin. She describes the teaching already given to Tom as *instruction*, that which *Tom simply needs to learn*. Her eager approach on this, wishing to see Tom recover as quickly as possible, has been noted in Tom's care notes. Nevertheless, Tom has only tentatively taken charge of his first injections. He seems reluctant to explore further what managing diabetes entails. Chloe, the specialist nurse, runs through the things that the ward staff have already 'briefed' Tom and Naomi about. *I say briefed,* she explains to them, *because I imagine that there was a lot to take in?* She learns that Tom has been told how insulin enables sugars to be used by cells but that in his condition there is a shortfall of insulin produced in his body. That is why insulin has to be injected. Tom knows that the insulin injection sites have to be changed in order to ensure a good uptake of the drug. The dose of his insulin is determined by the level of sugar to be 'mopped up' within his blood; that is why he has to prick his finger and test the blood sugar level. Tom admits to feeling vague about how all of this then relates to his diet.

Chloe notes how eager Naomi is about the mastery of self-care techniques. She appears to see this quite simply as a matter of mastering skills. Tom, though, pulls a face as he talks

(Continued)

(Continued)

about injecting himself with a drug. He seems uncertain about being dependent upon it and he quickly admits to being frightened about what might happen if he doesn't take his medication or else he gets the dosage of insulin wrong. He seems much less confident about managing his illness than his mother does.

Table 5.3 Principal steps in conducting a demonstration

Step	Notes
Create a private space and explain to the patient what you hope to demonstrate to them. Assure them that instant mastery is not assumed; you will guide them as required.	You need to establish a safe learning environment. Patients usually dislike the idea of performing a skill in front of onlookers other than their instructor. The emphasis is on exploration, a gradual enquiry into what can be achieved this time or perhaps over a number of repetitions.
Outline what you will do and explain why it is important to their care. Explain that you will talk through a complete explanation of the procedure so that they understand your reasoning as you go. Assure the patient that they can ask any questions that occur to them.	You must not assume patient consent to the procedure or the invitation to learn through a demonstration. Make sure that your explanation uses accessible language. Avoid complex medical terms if possible. Explain that you are interested in how the procedure feels, seems, as well as why it is important that it works. You reassure the patient that they retain control in this matter and can stop if alarmed.
Complete the procedure by talking aloud about your reasoning for each action as you go. Once you have completed the entire demonstration, explain how you will now review it in steps once again. With invasive measures such as injections you don't repeat the procedure immediately but you rehearse with the patient what you did first, second, third, etc. and why.	Patients need to first gain an overview of the procedure, from start to finish (e.g. self-injecting insulin). This enables them to understand how elements fit together. Patients typically fear that they will forget something, about the sequencing of steps, so that is why you will then break the procedure down into explained stages.
Check what the patient understands now about the procedure and assess how confident or apprehensive they are concerning it. If they express some confidence, negotiate how they can start to take charge next. That may entail them simply providing the running commentary to what you do. But if they are more confident, then they may complete the first steps of the procedure under your supervision.	The patient needs to draw breath and decide whether the procedure seems daunting. It is tempting at this stage to prompt them to immediate action, but resist that. You need to assure them that they can approach control of the procedure in a manageable way. Learning is an emotional enquiry and as a person-centred care nurse you are alert to their perceptions and feelings.

Step	Notes
Provide regular supportive feedback to the patient as they try out the procedural steps. Assure them that this doesn't have to be hurried, that you know they feel nervous. Explain that you will prevent them from taking any incorrect action.	What we take for granted is entirely new to the patient. Hands may shake when drawing up insulin. They may fear that the needle will be inserted at the wrong angle. They may fear that it hurts more, causing them to jag the needle out again. So reassure the patient about what they are doing right, show them how to position equipment appropriately.
Encourage the patient to review what they discovered at each step along the way. How did that feel? What did they notice? What seemed easy and what seemed hard about that step of the procedure?	Typically patients experience relief with each mastered step, so give them time to express their thoughts. But they may discover that the procedure is still difficult for them, so stand ready to applaud progress for now and agree that their attempt at the next stages can be arranged next time.
Congratulate the patient on what they have understood and achieved, no matter how hesitant the step taken. Highlight what you will refine or improve upon together next time.	Help the patient take stock and savour what they have now begun to control. Highlight how empowering this can be in the long term. Acknowledge any outstanding doubts and answer questions that they have. You will still supervise them at the next procedure, but perhaps that time, you will ask them to talk aloud about the reasoning for each step.

Activity 5.3   Reflection

Study the case of Tom now, and reflect upon what you know about family-centred care; the focus upon, in this instance, both Tom and Naomi. Do you think that son and mother have the same needs here? What do you think that might mean for the facilitation of learning to come?

An outline answer is given at the end of this chapter.

Anticipating patient care

In this case study Chloe draws upon a mix of evidence and experience to help her negotiate care with a patient such as Tom and his mother. The evidence is centred upon diabetes and how it represents a challenge to patients. There is some additional evidence related to learning to manage diabetes mellitus, but that is much less extensive than about the illness itself. Managing the dynamics of family-centred care and expressing that too, Chloe draws from extensive experience of working with different clients. For example, she appreciates that a parent is a potential colleague who cares for and might help teach a child diabetes management, but that relies upon assessing their grasp of the medical problem and what teaching activities are meant to achieve. If parent and nurse work from different premises, if they have different expectations of learning, then friction can quickly arise. Critical, then, to any future teaching work with Tom, it is necessary to ascertain whether Chloe can establish a rapport with Naomi and they can agree together with Tom a teaching plan that addresses all the different requirements.

Practice tip

Listen carefully to how a parent or other lay carer describes their child's illness and the challenges it poses. Perhaps that is a conversation you overhear amongst parents. The point is, your understanding of narrative doesn't always have to come from interview. Some insights are freely shared in other conversations.

Diabetes mellitus

Tom suffers from Type 1 diabetes mellitus. Diabetes mellitus is a condition affecting the metabolism of blood glucose so that it can be utilised within cells as a source of energy, or turned into fat deposits to be stored within depot areas of the body. Sugars are derived through foodstuffs (notably carbohydrates) and rendered amenable to use by body cells through the production of insulin in the pancreas. In Type 1 diabetes mellitus the beta cells of the pancreas are progressively destroyed as part of an auto-immune response. Why patients develop this form of diabetes remains unclear, but it has been postulated that both genetic and perhaps viral trigger factors play a part (Pearce, 2014). The net result of the destruction of the beta cells is that less and less insulin is available to process and reduce the level of blood sugar. Type 1 diabetes mellitus is most commonly associated with children or young adults (Scheiner, 2020).

Type 2 diabetes mellitus, in contrast, is not an auto-immune condition but poses a significant threat to the health of millions. The incidence of Type 1 diabetes mellitus is much less, accounting for around 10 per cent of diagnosed cases. However, because it has onset in early life and is not open to cure, it poses a lifelong self-treatment challenge for the patient (see Table 5.4).

Activity 5.4   Critical thinking

As Table 5.4 indicates, the medical problem is a relatively complex one. Imagine now that you are trying to summarise it for a parent such as Naomi. How might you characterise it?

An outline answer is given at the end of this chapter.

Table 5.4 Challenges that a patient diagnosed with Type 1 diabetes mellitus faces (the medical problem)

Problem	Notes
To control the level of dietary glucose intake (principally through controlled consumption of carbohydrates).	A patient with diabetes still needs a diet commensurate with their lifestyle energy demands, but this must be managed so as to match what subcutaneous insulin injections can help process.
To self-administer the right amount of insulin at the right times and in the right form so as to manage the level of blood glucose within target range.	Insulin is administered in different forms – short-, medium- and long-acting – in different combinations and times so as to manage the metabolic demands of the body at different times of the day and night, and to match mealtimes when glucose intake may increase. While target blood glucose levels are agreed with the patient, it is rare for these to be achieved and sustained perfectly day in, day out over the longer term (Pearce, 2014).
To re-evaluate lifestyle demands so that the right balance of glucose intake and insulin use is arrived at, adjusting the same according to periodic changes.	Young people vary their lifestyle, for example the balance of sleep and waking, time between meals, and they may make extra demands on blood glucose regulation, for instance when stressed or unwell. For that reason the balance of carbohydrate intake and insulin cannot remain a constant.
To ensure that the self-administered insulin is absorbed effectively.	The rate at which insulin is absorbed subcutaneously varies, with a slower and uneven absorption from sites used repeatedly for injection. So injection sites need to be changed. The patient might use an injection portal or an insulin pump to better regulate the supply of insulin.
To monitor for acute risks linked to an imbalance of too much insulin for too little glucose ingested (hypoglycaemia).	The most acute and potentially life-threatening risk is where a patient becomes hypoglycaemic and may collapse. Patients need to carry emergency sugar supply in the form of sweets. Patients learn to recognise early signs of hypoglycaemia.
To monitor for ongoing risks associated with inadequately controlled blood sugar levels (too much glucose in the blood) that leads to ketoacidosis, lethargia, loss of consciousness and increased risks of long-term systemic complications.	Multiple risks attend an inadequately controlled blood glucose level (hyperglycaemia), including damage to the heart, kidneys, eyes, limb circulation and brain. However, chronic, low-level hyperglycaemia may not register significantly as symptoms, making it easier for the patient to ignore that which is dangerous.
To re-evaluate self as someone who manages health in a more strategic and conscious way, managing that which did not require attention before.	Patients become people with diabetes, although in terms of owning the responsibilities for self-care they need to accept that they are diabetic. They must consciously manage their health in ways that other young people don't find a need to do.

Teaching patients about diabetes and its management

Chloe has personal experience of teaching individual patients, children, young people and older adults about diabetes mellitus and self-care, but she is aware as well of research that has been done into arranging education in different ways. Sometimes, one-to-one teaching is not necessarily the only or indeed the best way to teach a patient. For example, some individuals associate learning with being a member of a group, just like in school.

Diabetes education has often been arranged as a short course. In the Desmond Project (Developing Quality Structured Education in Diabetes, Desmond Project, 2018) learners receive six hours of teaching. In Denmark such learning may extend from a minimum of 10 hours of learning to over 24 hours of teaching conducted over 2 to 10 weeks (Laursen et al., 2017b). To make this cost-effective, learning is facilitated in groups. Patients complete a course of learning that attends not only to the illness of diabetes and its successful treatment, but also to lifestyle adjustment, for example diet and exercise.

Not all patients learn well in large groups, however (Grohmann et al., 2017), and there is a growing body of evidence relating to why patients do not attend self-care courses (Horigan et al., 2017). Patients may drop out, fearing comparison with their peers as well as because of logistical difficulties. Health coaching has been widely advocated as a way of helping patients to learn in a very person-centred way (Rogers and Maini, 2016). Coaching of this kind has developed apace since 2000 and it combines health education with health promotion. It combines shared goal setting with motivational interviewing, helping the patient to identify that which might best sustain healthy behaviours. The goal of health coaching is to enlighten the individual, but also to help them to act strategically, identifying obstacles to their chosen goals and ways to overcome them. However, because the learning is so one to one, and it may extend over a protracted period of time, it is costly to deliver.

Activity 5.5   Reflection

Think back to your own experience of learning and what seemed successful for you. Did you enjoy learning in a group and, if so, why? Did you prefer to learn privately with access to a tutor or other advisor; again, if so, why? What, when associated with an illness, might prompt you to either stick with your preferred form of learning or select another approach?

As this activity is based on your own reflection, no outline answer is provided at the end of the chapter.

Relating and person-centred care (assessing)

Chloe arranged to meet with both Tom and Naomi to better assess their needs and to establish how the diabetes management clinic could best help them. Rather than share a three-way conversation from the outset, though, she arranged for Naomi to arrive 30 minutes early for an opening conversation. Tom would then join them by taxi after he had finished school for the afternoon. Chloe chose this strategy because she said that Naomi had telephoned ahead early to press urgent points about what she felt might be required.

Had Chloe opened the discussion with Naomi and Tom together, she feared that she might not secure all perspectives on the health problem. As in other person-centred care, Chloe explained that she hoped to build rapport with both Tom and his mother, to further a trusting partnership that would in turn aid the plan of learning ahead of them. It would be necessary to listen attentively to each of her clients' narratives and to represent as clearly as possible what she hoped to offer them. Chloe said,

Nurses sometimes think that the only narrative is that of the patient or a relative, but we have narratives to share as well. If we hear only one narrative, then we fail. The medical problem demands that we add a narrative of our own. My narrative is really about three things. First, the need to actively manage the illness, it's a very important investment. Second, the need to fashion education that works for the patient. This isn't a formula. Third, the need to be patient and manage education in stages if necessary. It's an emotional challenge to understand and cope with diabetes.

I asked Chloe about whether she found that Naomi and her own narrative seemed in relative harmony at that first meeting. She admitted that they hadn't. There were some points of difference. First, Naomi was obviously an enthusiastic and very caring mother, but she had relatively firm views about dealing with illness. You analysed it and then you solved it. Naomi had not talked very much about the emotional dimension of the illness, confronting the need to treat yourself with insulin and control your diet for decades ahead. Second, Naomi was not entirely sure about what she called 'modern teaching methods' which she observed tended to 'tie students in knots'. There was 'something to be said for instruction', Naomi observed. She asked whether Chloe was planning to send Tom on a short course, alongside his peers. A 'brisk instruction' might achieve a good result. Chloe had agreed that this was an option; she taught on such a course herself. But it might also be beneficial to coach Tom. She asked whether Naomi felt comfortable with finding out about Tom's experiences and perceived needs before they decided altogether. Naomi agreed.

Next, Chloe asked whether Naomi saw herself teaching Tom as well. The question surprised Naomi. She had imagined that the nurses and therapists taught diabetes care. She would of course help with adjusting his diet and reminding him to monitor his blood sugar.

Do you expect me to teach? Naomi quizzed.

Not necessarily, Chloe assured her, some parents do and some don't. But it's good for us to identify what you would prefer now, so that we can work, each understanding what the other does. If we are comfortable with our roles, we can organise Tom's support. Learning diabetes self-care isn't like a lesson with homework, it's a constant demand on a boy, so I hope to help you in a way that makes sense from the beginning. What would you prefer, Naomi? Naomi said that she preferred not to teach and that it would seem better if she monitored how Tom was getting along with diabetes self-care. She would like to offer regular feedback to Chloe. Chloe said that was brilliant. No clinic visit could ever make up for monitoring in the home.

Practice tip

Clinical practice is likely to repeatedly present circumstances where a patient or relative raises expectations that surprise you. It's a good idea to note the same, draw breath and then consult with a colleague. Patients and relatives know that student nurses cannot instantly agree strategies. Use your learner status to appreciate with a colleague what is involved in patient requests or expectations.

Activity 5.6   Speculating

Pause now to speculate about what Chloe and Naomi's conversation was largely about. It included a review of best ways to cope or learn. But what else was it centring upon? Why was that important before Tom was invited to join the conversation?

An outline answer is given at the end of this chapter.

Chloe later said to me:

You think that I jumped the gun there, didn't you, planning roles when I'm still at the relating stage! But as we spoke I realised that Naomi thought very quickly about proper roles, proper techniques, and so it seemed likely to reassure her if I was equally direct about how we might work. Her narrative was about being rational, effective and business-like. So this time rapport building drew forward a discussion of roles. If I had shied away from that, then she wouldn't have thought me very convincing.

Tom joined the meeting and Chloe explained to me then how she gently explored his experiences to date. Using open questions, she encouraged him to 'think aloud how it had been'. Naomi watched intently how Chloe sustained eye contact with Tom, acknowledged his discomforts and jotted down what he said. Tom identified the following concerns:

1. Feeling dependent on insulin, which he referred to as a drug. People who used needles on themselves might be misunderstood as drug addicts.

2. Feeling anxious about rescue treatment, by which he meant emergency sugar intake or insulin. Chloe asked what these emergencies felt like and he admitted that he wasn't sure.

3. Needing to adjust the insulin in some way – perhaps the mix of types of insulin, and/or the volume of insulin taken in a day. Chloe asked if he meant when he did exercise, or perhaps had the flu. He said yes.

4. Stopping diabetes from 'wrecking' his body 'in the long run'.

Chloe then asked Naomi what she thought; did that seem a clear list of concerns to start with? She said that it did. Some had surprised Naomi, such as Tom's worries about what using a hypodermic needle signified. *You tell them that you're diabetic,* she said, *we tell the teachers so they can support you.*

Tom said, *you're grown-up, mum, my friends aren't. They don't understand like you.*

Chloe and I discussed what the list of Tom's perceptions, his early needs, meant for the next stage of work, negotiating a good way forward. We agreed that there was a hierarchy of concerns, at the top of which was his need to seem acceptable, normal, not a drug addict because he self-injected insulin. This wasn't the top-ranking medical problem – adequate and safe regulation of blood sugar was – but if Tom didn't get that personal image need addressed, he wouldn't feel confident about his forthcoming teaching. The next thing we agreed was that Tom knew diabetes in the abstract, as a kind of theory. He didn't know what risk felt like and because of that he couldn't be sure that rescue measures would readily work. Learning sometimes has to engage feelings as well as knowledge (Jones et al., 2019). The third thing that we agreed was that Tom wanted to be able to plan things. He wanted to be able to adjust his insulin therapy and he didn't know how. This encouraged us because Tom seemed motivated to understand. He said, *I want to boss it rather than it boss me.* Lastly, Tom understood that he would need to protect his body from harm 'in the long run', but this wasn't the most pressing problem right now.

I asked Chloe whether she thought Naomi might agree with that assessment and she explained:

Naomi wanted to give Tom the whole package immediately, to equip him with all he needed to know. She recognised the medical problem immediately and wanted to head that off. It would be how I might feel if I was a mother.

I asked her then what that meant for negotiating patient care.

Two things, said Chloe. *First I had to negotiate a case for taking things a step at a time, starting with Tom's worries. It didn't sound as though a diabetes short course would necessarily answer that. Second, it meant persuading Naomi to trust us while we tried out certain well-managed experiences to help build Tom's confidence.*

Activity 5.7   Critical thinking

At this point Chloe has begun to weave insights from both Naomi and Tom's narrative together. This process is called conceptualisation. We turn a series of points into something that encapsulates what they are all about. We name the problem or need. Naomi wants to protect her son and to counter diabetes as quickly as possible. Tom still wanted to develop

(Continued)

(Continued)

an account of himself and how he is coping. So Tom is tentatively exploring. See if you can guess now what this means for the following before you read on.

1. The design of Tom's teaching package.
2. The liaison work that Chloe will need to do with Naomi.
3. Reassuring Tom that he can cope effectively.

As the text below answers this activity, no outline answer is given at the end of the chapter.

Practice tip

Listening to patients or relatives speak about a problem or need, you can sometimes notice the way they return again and again to an issue. Just how much their attention centres upon a particular issue is a reasonable way to judge its importance. Attending to their worry quickly improves the chance that you build rapport with the patient.

Negotiating person-centred care (planning)

I felt that I could guess what Chloe might recommend to Tom and his mother. I believed that she would recommend some form of coaching rather than the two-day diabetes self-care course that the centre ran. The course was extremely good at delivering more information to participants and improving techniques such as self-injection, but it was a more one-size-fits-all provision. Further, a new course started every six weeks and it seemed likely that Naomi would expect Chloe to proceed apace with some kind of teaching.

Chloe smiled. She hoped to coach Tom in a new way, working with another diabetic patient, a 16-year-old teenager called Gina. She explained that if she coached Tom by herself that would be very resource intensive and there might be a growing pressure from Naomi to instruct more. Chloe said,

> I'd like to work with Gina and Tom together because I think it will make it easier to help him build a new account of who he is as a diabetic. It will reassure him that other teenagers cope well. Gina wants to become a diabetes mentor and she's already dealt with some worries that Tom might meet. But I think too that working that way can help Tom explore his control of the illness. His injection technique looked reasonably sound, but he needs to judge how to counter problems and protect himself from risks in the future.

Chloe presented both educational options to Tom and Naomi. Then she went on to explore the fit of each with Tom's expressed needs. She explained that she was proposing Gina as a mentor and suggested that they might start with a day that enabled Tom to hear about how Gina coped with becoming diabetic and which helped him to explore the management of risks. The three of them would spend the day together, go running in the park, and delay Tom's food intake so that he could experience hypoglycaemia in a very controlled way and then the beneficial effects of using glucose to combat that. She explained to Tom that she had some 'what if …' scenario cards that she wanted to share with them both and to then see if they could identify what problems might arise and what they could do about them.

> *I said to Tom that I wanted to work with him about how it felt to be diabetic, describing that to others, and it seemed a good idea to ask Gina to help with that. We will start with your first on the list concern, Tom. Then we will spend the rest of the day on building some confidence with anticipating and countering risks that can arise. I assured Tom that we would discuss managing the longer-term challenges of diabetes after that teaching day. The long-term challenges were real, but it was a good idea to build confidence with immediate worries first.*

I asked Chloe how that suggestion had been received and she explained that Naomi didn't want to wait for Tom to join a group course. If they had to wait, then they might set up some learning of their own, on the internet. Chloe responded that coaching would probably work very well. She had a limited budget of time for coaching but working with two patients rather than one made the venture more cost-effective.

Activity 5.8 Reflection

What do you think are the merits of the mentored teaching day for a patient such as Tom? Why might it be important for Tom to experience a problem (like carefully controlled hypoglycaemia) and to link the solutions to what a mentor like Gina could offer? What do you imagine might be the advantages of using 'what if …' scenario cards that challenged Tom and Gina alike?

An outline answer is given at the end of this chapter.

A teaching plan

Before we move on to collaborating, I want to offer points about a written plan. In this case the plan became a teaching strategy for the teaching day. You might wonder what such a plan looks like. If the patient and the nurse negotiate a plan together, what form does the record then take? Unless a registered nurse has completed a mentorship or clinical teaching course, it is unlikely that they are versed in writing teaching plans. So I asked Chloe to talk about the simple plan that she drafted with Tom. Did it look like a nursing care plan, one that worded the problem or need firmly in terms of Tom's perceptions, followed by response actions, rationale and planned completion date?

Chloe explained that she set out each of Tom's priority needs in simple form at the top of a page.

1. Need to explain my diabetes and treatment to others (she added a red dot)

2. Need to anticipate and manage short-term risks linked to diabetes and my treatment (she added a blue dot)

3. Need to be able to adjust my treatment to suit changing circumstances (she added a green dot).

Then she set out a series of planned sessions for the course of the day (a timetable) and she added the relevant coloured dot to each session. That would enable Tom to see that she was keeping the day properly focused on his concerns. To each of the sessions she added a note briefly describing what everyone would be doing. None of the sessions lasted for more than 60 minutes. She had scheduled in lunchtime for Gina and Tom to discuss diabetes privately, if they so wished. At the end of the day there would be a wash-up discussion to determine what had been learned and what was yet unclear or worrying. The sequence of sessions was as follows (Table 5.5).

Table 5.5   A teaching plan

Session	Notes
Introductions and Gina's story (red and blue dot)	Chloe asked Gina to talk first of all, enabling Tom to feel safe listening to Gina's story. He would be encouraged to ask questions at the end. Gina was asked to describe her experiences using her preferred analogy. She was a keen dinghy sailor and she likened the body to her boat, foodstuffs being the wind source. But for the food to aid the body, there had to be fine tuning of blood sugar, enabling it to enter the cells (the sail had to be trimmed). If the body had too much of one, then the body (Gina's boat) lost control. Gina was asked to explain how she had dealt with friends' enquiries and misunderstandings about diabetes, especially fears held by some of her peers that she might now be fragile.
Park run, feeling fit (blue and red dot)	After coffee (but no cake) Gina, Tom and Chloe to complete a park run next to the clinic. The purpose of this is both to talk about feeling fit and well, and also to facilitate a controlled fall in blood sugar. Tom and Gina will share a later lunch and explore how it feels to become mildly hypoglycaemic. Tom is to learn about the experience and realise just how quickly a sugar intake could rectify the problem. The three of them will discuss how that feels personally and also how it might be explained to friends.

Session	Notes
Lunch	Private discussion time for Gina and Tom
'What if …' scenario exercise (red, blue and green dots)	Tom and Gina are challenged with a series of 'what if …' scenario cards, describing different developments. Some are medical problems (e.g. developing a chest infection) and some are more personal problems (for example, explaining to a curious peer the content of your medical equipment bag). The purpose of the session is to help both learners see themselves as problem solvers, building confidence through development of a shared set of answers. Chloe plays the role of agent provocateur. ('But what if your friend kept pestering you with questions, about whether you could ever go away somewhere there wasn't a refrigerator for insulin, for instance?')
Strategic management of living with diabetes (blue and green dots)	Chloe provides a briefing on the strategic planning of lifestyle and medication, showing how life can be planned and treatment adjusted. She will show them different insulins, discuss what an insulin pump can do and discuss the pros and cons of different ways of supplying the insulin. This session will emphasise strategy, the merit of keeping a diary in case the patient wants to ask for a change in their diabetes treatment regime. Helping doctors and nurses to understand a need is important and could give Tom or Gina greater control.
Wash-up evaluation	What have we learned? What still seems missing or worrying? What was successful and less successful about the learning arrangements? Do we want to stay in touch to discuss future diabetes issues?

What is important about the design of this teaching day is that it centres so clearly on Tom's expressed needs. It also addresses Gina's objectives about becoming a mentor, but that is beyond the scope of our case study here. Tom moves from a start of relatively passive learning (he listens to Gina) to a role of problem solving alongside her. Chloe is acutely aware of the need for Tom to develop confidence learning with another person. He needs to feel, if not expert, then capable of making a useful contribution, so the problem-solving session occurs later in the day when he knows Gina rather better. The day is based on discovery and experience. The most formal teaching by Chloe (an explanation of insulin and delivery arrangements) occurs at the end of the day. This, Chloe explains, helps patients to feel that they drive decisions. Would some of this help me? What would I like to do? It would be relatively easier to deliver the content of this day by simply lecturing Tom and Gina side by side, but that would be to miss the point; learning to manage diabetes involves understanding your own experiences and finding responses that *you* are confident about.

Practice tip

The form that care or teaching plans take may vary markedly dependent on the care environment and circumstances prevailing there. There is no set format for such plans. But you can check whether they are person-centred by:

(Continued)

(Continued)

- noting whether they relate to perceptions that you have heard the patient voice;
- determining whether the plan has changed pace or direction with regard to a patient-expressed concern;
- checking who has access to the plan (logically patients should be able to access records that capture what they contribute to).

Collaborating on person-centred nursing care (implementing)

One of the things that the teaching plan does is highlight a design for learning. It imagines what the learners are going to do, in what order and to what purpose. The teaching that you will be engaged in might be less complex than what Chloe does as a Clinical Nurse Specialist, but it can still involve elements of design. There may, for example, be a planned use of measurement, the patient perhaps evaluating incremental wound closure. The teacher enables the student to not only achieve particular skills but also to sense progress, to feel increasingly able to carry on learning after teaching has concluded. Just as person-centred care empowers the person, so too does a student-centred facilitation-of-learning approach. In mental health, a diary might be used to help a patient realise just how rare angry outbursts have become; how they are now better able to countenance difficulties in daily living. The nurse imagines how an activity will help the learner feel as well as what it will ask them to do.

I was curious, however, to learn from Chloe what teaching, or, more accurately here, coaching (a form of one-to-one or very small group teaching), involved. What did she actually do on the day? What did coaching entail? We sat down and pieced together the following features of the day.

Realising, not telling

Chloe explained that it is very tempting for a Clinical Nurse Specialist to spend a lot of her time telling other people about what experts know. After all, the job title implies a certain expertise. It is gratifying to secure quick thanks from patients or relatives, based on how much information you are able to convey in a short space of time. But Chloe's deep conviction was that if people try things for themselves, rather than simply listen to information, then they secure a deeper and more sustained kind of learning. To that end, during the day she resisted the temptation to explain everything immediately, before Tom and Gina had time to explore ideas and solutions of their own. Chloe believed that they would derive a great deal more satisfaction from discovery.

I suggested to Chloe that teaching required patience and the conviction that you were making a difference. Your work wasn't measured by the number of slides shown to a patient or the number of handouts supplied. What seemed particularly valuable was the use of Gina's narrative of illness and coping at the start of the day. In person-centred care the narrative was pivotal too (see Chapter 2) and there was no reason why a patient might not learn something from someone else's narrative. Learners understood things, though, to the extent that you helped them to linger on a point before rushing on. So, when Tom stopped to ask whether Gina handled diabetes differently, being a girl, Chloe was able to help out. She reminded them that could be important in two ways. First, did others behave differently to you as a diabetic, because you were female? But it could also be an issue relating to body differences, menstrual periods; it was possible that cyclic changes within the body might complicate self-care. Chloe quickly assured Gina that there was no need to discuss her private health to that degree, but Gina was keen to answer honestly. She sometimes had heavy periods and that affected her energy and confidence. So she felt the need to be 'on top of diabetes all of the time'. Tom had listened intently, respectfully, and later explained how disciplined and determined Gina had seemed. Listening to her, he felt that you could manage your life despite diabetes.

Activity 5.9   Reflection

What have been your working assumptions about teaching? Do you imagine that teachers always talk a lot? Do they instead listen effectively in order to ask questions and make suggestions at different points? Does this in turn help you believe that you might be able to teach as well, in some carefully targeted, modest way?

An outline answer is given at the end of this chapter.

Listening intently

Chloe explained that setting learning exercises such as the 'what if …' scenarios was certainly not a lazy form of teaching. She had to interpret quickly and accurately what Gina and Tom were saying. Even chat whilst running in the park was not entirely social. Chloe explained that she attended to everything that the others said and the way that they said it. For example, Tom expressed doubts about what diabetes might enable him to do. He felt out of breath quite quickly even though before becoming ill he had been a school football team player. For Chloe this suggested a doubt about remaining extremely fit and diabetic. So as they ran, she thought about sportsmen and women who she knew were diabetic and had excelled. Then at the end of the run she asked Tom what the sport celebrities all had in common. He immediately guessed that they were all diabetic. 'More than that?!' Chloe challenged. Tom didn't know, but Gina did; each of the athletes had met injury or other illness setbacks that temporarily stalled their careers. They had needed to manage diabetes through that as well. Resilience could be learned, Chloe suggested, if you understood your illness and responded very well indeed. Notice the parallel here: the importance of listening attentively in person-centred care and, if you are coaching someone, to believe in them.

Drawing down on experience

I asked Chloe whether she quoted research evidence to Tom and Gina as part of her coaching and she observed that no, that was kept in the background unless patients asked for such material. It was motivating for some. What was important, though, was to draw down on her experience of helping other patients. So in the 'what if ...' scenario session and the explanation of uses of different forms of insulin she had regularly referred to past patient experiences of managing problems. Each of the examples was rendered anonymous (she didn't name individual patients) but she observed that such experience seemed powerful and authentic for learners irrespective of how young or old they were. The more similar other patients' situations were to the current patient's concern, the more powerful was the shared story of coping.

Activity 5.10   Critical thinking

Have you deployed experience, anecdotal stories of what other patients have met or done to manage a health problem? Do you think that there are important rules to follow when teaching with such information?

An outline answer is given at the end of this chapter.

Rewarding and celebrating

It might be easy to caricature coaching as a wildly enthusiastic form of teaching, one where the teacher is almost evangelical about the process and what has been achieved. Chloe insisted that this shouldn't be overdone as that tended to convey a desperate desire for the teaching to be appreciated. If you overdid the celebration of discovery, it might say more about your teaching feedback needs. Instead, what was better was a carefully focused series of positive appraisals during the course of the day, identifying what the patient/learner had achieved. The same should always be linked to an invite for someone like Tom to share their own judgement on progress. Chloe said,

> I admit it, I wanted Tom to be able to go home to Naomi and report what a great day of learning he had just enjoyed. I wanted it to be impressive. But what was more important was for the day to give enough reward to sustain Tom's motivation and to enable him to understand how his reasoning was changing.

I asked Chloe to clarify her remark about reasoning. She explained that the day was about helping him to think differently, to believe that he could have greater charge of his health circumstances. It was about realising that he could discover things for himself and convey his needs comfortably to others. Chloe's rewarding then consisted of regular, carefully observed remarks on progress made. The comments centred on what seemed to have been discovered and why that might be valuable in the future. Chloe, for example, remarked during the 'what if …' scenario session on how Tom seemed comfortable debating aloud different responses to problems that might arise. If there was a heavy reliance on just one solution, then a patient might find it harder to manage their diabetes under a range of new circumstances. Imagining different ways to solve a problem increased options for the future – and perhaps that created a feeling of greater freedom? Chloe let the question linger with Tom. *Yes,* he agreed with a smile.

Practice tip

A good way to start teaching is to operate in pairs, each nurse helping the patient to explore the subject in hand. One nurse explains chosen points whilst the second carefully observes patient response. The second nurse then helps the patient to explore any concerns or questions that have arisen. Now the first nurse observes what ensues before returning to the next explanations to be shared. Whilst this is initially resource intensive, it should help you develop confidence in your ability to exercise one or more teaching components discussed in this chapter.

Evaluating person-centred care (evaluating)

Chloe proposed to Tom and Gina that everyone should rehearse aloud what had seemed valuable and less than useful about the teaching day, and then to identify what might yet need to be dealt with. Gina and Tom had talked comfortably during the day so this 360-degree review, including an invite to comment on how the day had been organised and run, seemed a possibility to Chloe. Tom and Gina were reluctant to begin, however, even though Chloe had encouraged them to be frank.

Chloe said she felt that the day had focused accurately on an important need, to explore ways of representing diabetes to other people. It had seemed to centre on creating positive impressions of healthy living. There were enthusiastic nods from both participants. But, Chloe continued, *in the last session I rather slid into explaining complications of uncontrolled levels of high blood sugar, didn't I? I was going to discuss that with you, Tom, later on. I wondered whether that confused the information about using insulin in different ways?*

Tom said that this may be the case. The need to manage diabetes in different ways was important for morale now. Avoiding long-term complications was important but perhaps that changed the feel of the teaching. *It sounded more 'you must',* he observed shyly, *when the rest of the session was 'here's how!'*

Activity 5.11 Reflection

What do you think about criticising yourself as the teacher or coach in this way? Do you think it has a clear purpose? Is evaluation solely about performance or is it equally about discovery in person-centred forms of care?

An outline answer is given at the end of this chapter.

Tom observed that the day had been a success because he could explain to himself and to his mother how he wanted to handle diabetes issues. It was about discovering what he wanted to say as well as about self-medication. The demonstrations in the hospital, how to test your own blood and give yourself an injection, had been about meeting the demands of the illness. There had been little time to discuss what he wanted to do. Whilst the illness 'made you do things to stay alive', there was a need to learn about feeling okay as well. You needed to feel that you had a say in coping. Tom paid Gina a compliment, saying that she had helped him believe that he could manage enquiries at school. Tom now planned to return to football training again. Chloe smiled. It was a very encouraging accolade for Gina, who wanted to mentor others.

Gina's evaluation was crisp and incisive. She explained how you forgot things; about how bewildering diabetes seemed at first. The risk then was that you were too brusque in advising others how to solve problems. Tom assured her that she hadn't seemed brusque at all. Nonetheless, Gina assured him, *I had to think hard about why you asked some questions, to imagine again how you were feeling.* There was a risk of thinking in a short-hand way to suggest solutions, rather than exploring how something felt.

Interestingly, the wash-up discussion centred on satisfaction with contributions made by each of the three parties involved. It was fairly performance-centred. I asked Chloe whether Tom had explored what yet seemed to be learned. Chloe admitted that he had not, although she had a scheduled meeting with him for later the next week. Perhaps he might take stock then? I asked about Naomi's evaluation of the service as she was a stakeholder too. Chloe explained that she had telephoned Naomi three days after the teaching day to ascertain if there were insights to be gained there. Naomi described how much less tense Tom now seemed. He seemed to be more confident about issues that might arise. At the end of the conversation Naomi thanked Chloe for her help and said that she was sorry if she had sounded abrupt when they first met. She had realised that when problems arose she was often hypercritical of services. So a garage might undergo 'my gimlet eye', she explained, because she didn't trust things to go smoothly after a car breakdown. *I become pretty sharp*, Naomi said. Chloe said that diabetes was stressful and not just for a child. Sometimes parents didn't know how they would react. Nurses simply did what they could to help them.

Person-centred care insights

I hope that one of the first insights you gained from this case study is how remarkably similar person-centred care and facilitated learning are to one another. Both begin with an understanding of the patient's narrative, the account of perceptions. Both person-centred care and facilitated learning are concerned with helping the individual to make sense of their experiences (Price, 2015). Getting better and learning involve an emotional as well as a skill development journey. Whilst there are forms of teaching (for instance, some lectures) that might seem rather more instructional, coaching in particular represents a psychological support. If you look back to Table 5.1, I think you might decide that it engaged a range of teaching elements to strategic purpose. If you have an instinct to explain, to guide and to support, then you start with an advantage when it comes to teaching. You are likely to be acutely aware of how your help is received and used by the patient. In this case Chloe monitored both Tom and Gina closely during the course of the teaching day. She was more interested in learning than teaching and whilst at the end she worried about overextending the last session, she was very encouraged by how both patients talked about self-care.

I want to suggest to you that this should give you encouragement to believe that you can contribute modest teaching as well. Whilst people complete lengthy courses on the theory and practice of education, curriculum development and design, some useful precepts can be learned quite quickly and with modest education. Coaching in particular, in its simplest form, becomes a purposeful form of helping. An amateur football coach (I did such a course) is not a lengthy affair and it centres as much on sustaining and motivating learners as well as teaching particular skills. Chloe brought to such coaching her experience of how other patients had responded to the help that she gave. She also deployed her imagination, pausing to reflect on how she would like to learn if she was confronted with a chronic illness.

Chloe said to me, I kept asking you during that day what theory supported what I was doing and you encouraged me to trust experience as well. That was true, I had encouraged her to work with instinct and experience. I asked her, What encourages Tom to trust your exercises and activities? She answered, He thinks that I want him to succeed. Yes, trust was important. Next I said to her, When you teach it's best to move from the known to the unknown and from something easier to something harder; is your teaching day designed like that? She agreed that it was. The day started with experience and not too many difficult demands. It had progressively become more demanding. Whilst I could harness a theory of learning to that, I suggested to her that equally compelling might be her experience of sustaining hope. First, you must convince the patient that you are interested in their needs. Next, you must help them believe that they can creep up on more daunting challenges by reducing the difficulty a step at a time. So even without an educational theory, a person-centred instinct, empathy and experience of how others seemed to learn best could carry the nurse a considerable way.

Teaching in this sense is not primarily to do with a written plan, the formulation of objectives or complex assessment techniques. The teaching plan was very simple indeed. I rather like the colour-dot system linking a teaching session to Tom's stated needs. Some of the sessions could reasonably address more than one of those. What is required is a methodical enquiry into where the patient/learner starts from. In this case study, that involved a willingness to clarify the different expectations of the patient and his parent. It would have been relatively easy to conflate the two narratives and for perhaps Naomi's to possibly dominate the support that Chloe then provided. Instead, though, Chloe stood her ground, adding a narrative of her own about what seemed to work well in helping patients master diabetes self-care. She clarified at the outset which role Naomi felt able to fulfil and then explored with Tom what it might feel like to be coached on a teaching day.

Chapter summary

Whilst not all person-centred care involves teaching, where it does it offers the potential to reach inside a person's life and to help them to refashion it in a way that seems valuable to the individual. Teaching empowers patients where it is designed well and where it centres on the business of learning, rather than exposition: the proving of nurse teacher expertise. Teaching should be the humble servant of patient rehabilitation.

In this chapter I have explained how one patient was assisted to build confidence and self-esteem through a teaching day, one that artfully met the needs of another patient called Gina. Teaching, like care, has to be negotiated and in this instance that meant reassuring Naomi, Tom's mother, that the strategy might prove beneficial. In child health and children's nursing there are a variety of stakeholders and a potential to cast parents and others as care collaborators or teaching companions. When a person-centred nurse teaches well, he or she sometimes demonstrates considerable powers of diplomacy as well as of psychological support.

Activities: Brief outline answers

Activity 5.2 Critical thinking (p104)

I think that the most obvious question is whether or not the patient seems capable and ready to concentrate on learning about their condition and its management. We should not presume that all patients are motivated to learn. Some patients may be too stressed, confused or shocked to respond to our teaching efforts. In acute-care nursing you are not usually required to undertake a comprehensive assessment of the patient's intellect, their level of reasoning, but you do need to attend to the way that they describe their circumstances. That will provide clues about their level of understanding and what they imagine solutions to the problem might entail. In acute care the medical problem sometimes drives a teaching imperative, to ensure that the patient masters at least some self-care measures before they are discharged from hospital. But even in that circumstance it is wise to acknowledge an ongoing educational need and to refer the patient to other teaching support when they are better equipped to make use of that.

Activity 5.3 Reflection (p107)

I think that Tom and Naomi may have quite separate and not necessarily complementary needs here. Naomi needs reassurance that the threat of illness can be quickly countered for her son and she seems to believe that this requires his instruction. It is tempting to imagine that such expectations are naïve, even ignorant, because learning takes time, but we shouldn't underestimate how illness threatens a parent as well. Tom's needs are arguably less clear but more centred on making sense of how best to cope with diabetes. He is still working out his own needs. For that reason it will be necessary to pause the urgently felt needs of Naomi to accommodate the exploration-of-illness needs of Tom. This will require considerable tact.

Activity 5.4 Critical thinking (p108)

My own approach here is to start simply. If the relative or patient is more inquisitive, I might draw diagrams on paper, but I start simply and see how far they want to go first. So diabetes mellitus Type 1 is the problem of keeping the body supplied with fuel in a properly regulated way. Cells need sugar for energy but if the patient produces no insulin, then sugar cannot be absorbed into the cells. The sugar remains in the bloodstream and can cause a lot of future problems to our body organs. So we need to replace the missing body insulin with that which we inject. Our replacement insulin isn't as evenly supplied as that from the body itself, so we have to monitor how it is reducing excess blood sugar. Our replacement system approximates what the body does and we have to learn techniques about how to manage that deftly.

Activity 5.6 Speculating (p112)

This conversation is about sorting out agendas and about finding a way to collaborate. Both Naomi and Chloe wish to see Tom benefit from the clinic, but that is only possible if parent and nurse agree roles and responsibilities and expertise is acknowledged. There is a potential for conflict here and a need to establish trust. Parents cannot instantly assess the nurse's expertise; the practitioner's experience is not printed on her sleeve, nor does a title or qualification necessarily assure a worried parent. So the nurse has to find ways to acknowledge parental fears and to create sufficient space for the problem to be assessed. As a 14-year-old, Tom becomes a very equal partner in care planning, but it might be unwise to unravel competing agendas of parent and son in a three-way conversation. Chloe does not know how Tom and Naomi relate to each other. Understanding the perceptions of a parent first can sometimes help care plan negotiation.

Activity 5.8 Reflection (p115)

A cost–benefit analysis of the teaching day might raise objections as regards the teaching time spent versus number of beneficiaries equation, but that makes assumptions about education measured as volume of information conveyed to an audience. A better equation might relate to long-term, sustained command of an illness or deficit that could counter expensive correction of problems in the future. I believe that Chloe has found a viable solution for Tom, who needs to be convinced that he can cope well and convey his new coping to others later on. A teenager might be more persuaded to embrace a challenge if a peer role-models successful coping too. Tom is likely to experience periodic hypoglycaemia for a variety of reasons but it seems better to know that he can tackle it quickly and effectively through a controlled experience. Tom will need to brief others who might have to help him, so confidence is important. 'What if …' scenarios, each printed on a card, are a good way to encourage discussion and shared problem solving. It is an approach to learning that works well in developing confidence about personal ability, something that is important for diabetics.

Activity 5.9 Reflection (p119)

Professional teachers are much more interested in learning and what evokes that. But it is common for the wider public to see teaching as a technique; a trick or an ability to instruct students. We certainly need some good technique but most people, parents, mentors, friends, guides, youth leaders, sports leaders, teach in some way at some time. So teaching isn't a strange activity; it is something that nurses can develop incrementally from a base as they explain and advise patients. One of your best portfolio long-term skill development activities could usefully centre on teaching.

Activity 5.10 Critical thinking (p120)

In my experience nurses often use anecdotes to help patients cope with or solve health problems. Sometimes that stems from the nurse's analysis of what they might do themselves. But we do need to emphasise in such circumstances that we are using anecdotes to help someone reason issues for themselves. We are not prescribing a solution. Patients might search for additional evidence; we might refer them to people with additional expertise. Teaching certainly draws upon experience, but we need a touch of humility regarding that.

Activity 5.11 Reflection (p122)

In this instance Chloe role-models evaluation, starting with her own work. In healthcare the evaluative tradition has tended to centre on performance review. There is nothing wrong with that provided that it is contextual; we remember the conditions under which we practise. Here Chloe uses the approach to very clear purpose, encouraging Tom and Gina to be honest and searching in their review. I'm not entirely sure that it is successful as each tended to review their own performance. A complementary review might have centred more on learning; what was discovered.

Further reading

Bastable, S (2017) *Essentials of Patient Education*, 5th edition. London: Jones and Barkett Publishers.

Bastable offers an accessible and wide-ranging guide to the principles of teaching and learning that you can dip into and utilise in a variety of contexts.

Mertig, R (2012) *Nurses' Guide to Teaching Diabetes Self-Management*, 2nd edition. New York: Springer.

Diabetes management regimens move on apace, but this book still offers good advice on teaching principles.

Morris, N (2020) *Find Your Way: A Story and Drama Resource to Promote Mental Wellbeing in Young People*. Shoreham-by-Sea: Pavilion Publishing.

This is an interesting resource which draws heavily on narrative, story and anecdote to promote mental health. It offers a series of case study stories that might serve well in clinical practice.

Rollnick, S, Miller, W and Buttler, C (2008) *Motivational Interviewing in Healthcare: Helping Patients Change Behaviour*. New York: The Guilford Press.

Motivational interviewing draws on both the psychology of counselling and of learning, and it represents a practical illustration of how learning can be facilitated on a one-to-one basis.

Useful websites

An interesting exercise is to visit several websites that offer teaching on the management of a condition. Next, determine how teaching seems to be conceived of there (see Table 5.1 in this chapter). What scope exists for people managing a condition to add to the teaching package, perhaps to share their coping recommendations? How is learning conceived of there – as an investigative process or something designed to quickly reassure? Below is a sample of websites to get you started.

www.arthritis.org

www.breastcancer.org

www.diabetes.co.uk/how-to/control-diabetes.html

www.moodjuice.Scot.nhs.uk/anxiety.asp

Teaching online via a website poses a new set of challenges, for instance checking what the patient understands or feels comfortable with. The easiest thing for organisations running websites to do is simply to supply information, but teaching is a little more than that. As you may in the future recommend such sites to patients, though, it seems a good idea to characterise what seems best in a teaching approach.

Chapter 6 Case study four

Helping Susan counter depression

NMC Future Nurse Standards of Proficiency for Registered Nurses

This chapter will address the following platforms and proficiencies:

Platform 1: Being an accountable professional

At the point of registration, the registered nurse will be able to:

1.9 understand the need to base all decisions regarding care and interventions on people's needs and preferences, recognising and understanding any personal and external factors that may unduly influence your decisions.

1.12 demonstrate the skills and abilities required to support people at all stages of life who are emotionally or physically vulnerable.

1.18 demonstrate the knowledge and confidence to contribute effectively and pro-actively in an interdisciplinary team.

Chapter aims

After reading this chapter, you will be able to:

- critically examine the ways in which the nurse might work with a patient and others to personalise the support of a patient with a mental illness;
- demonstrate further awareness regarding the need for clinicians to revisit previous care interventions and to think again about future options.

Introduction

The case study chapters of this book have explored care at evolving stages of the professional relationship, and I have now moved beyond rehabilitation and into the realms of self-care and health maintenance. Here, too, it is important to make care personal, working closely with the patient's circumstances. In the first case studies that you have read, the medical problem loomed large, setting imperatives that had to be addressed. There, person-centred care often focuses on understanding the demand posed by illness and finding ways to respond to it. In severe Covid-19 infection the need for oxygen and assisted respiration may be indisputable, just as the need to inject insulin dominates the circumstances of a Type 1 diabetic. Some measures are imperative. In this case study, though, we move to a situation where the personal problem is the major challenge and where different treatment options might have a clearer role to play. Now there is greater scope for the patient to negotiate decisions and because they deal with illness over the longer term, they have insights of their own to bring to the care negotiation.

In this chapter I would like you to pay particular attention to the way that Gillian (the nurse) and Stewart (the GP) draw on different evidence, learning lessons from the past and adjusting care with Susan (the patient) for the future. This case study is closely associated with motivating a patient, something that recurs as a challenge in person-centred care. To succeed, patients must want to be our partners and want to sustain their health over time. To that end, nurses have to consider how best to enthuse patients, finding common purpose in the care shared. Without an understanding of human motivation, it is very hard to build on the benefits of care to date.

Depression

Mind (2018) observes that one in six people in England will suffer mental health problems, such as depression or anxiety, within their lifetime. Depression is the leading cause of disability worldwide (Pols et al., 2017), with 615 million people suffering from this condition (Counselling Directory, 2018). NICE (2009) observes that adult depression has a high relapse rate, with patients suffering repeat bouts of depression during the course of their lifetime. For that reason, self-care and motivation remain vitally important.

Depression may arise in association with clear co-morbidities (such as diabetes mellitus or coronary artery disease) or it may arise in ambiguous circumstances. NICE guidelines (2009) make it clear that, while a stepped approach to management is preferred (with medication reserved for more severe cases), successful treatments may be highly dependent on the patient's personal circumstances. What works well for one patient might not succeed with another. Treatment might focus upon:

- adjustments to the environment (for example, light therapy to counter seasonal affective disorder) (Kragh et al., 2017);
- chemical adjustments within the brain secured by antidepressants (Anderson and Tapesh, 2013) or electroconvulsive therapy (ECT) (Leaver et al., 2018);
- learning new coping behaviours (cognitive behavioural therapy) (Conklin and Strunk, 2015);
- understanding and countering negative emotions (Counselling for Depression (CfD)) (Goldman et al., 2016);
- more explorative measures such as vagal stimulation (Feldman et al., 2013) and acupuncture (Hopton et al., 2014).

That depression admits of a range of possible treatments, often used in combination, and that NICE (2009) acknowledges that significant further research is still needed signals that negotiating best treatment, sustaining patient motivation and keeping them well represent significant challenges for nurses.

Nurses need to understand what motivates a patient to sustain behaviours that minimise the risk of relapse. In depression, this is difficult. One of the cardinal symptoms of depression is that patients lose hope. Depression is a condition characterised by:

- depressed mood;
- lost interest/pleasure in activities;
- low energy levels;
- feelings of low self-worth or guilt;
- negativity or feelings of helplessness;
- disturbed sleep and/or appetite (Sanders and Hill, 2014; Murphy, 2019).

Therefore, working with motivation is a key concern for the nurse. Recourse to antidepressant medication is rarely the complete solution. The Royal College of Psychiatrists (2009) observes that only 50–65 per cent of patients respond to medication, that the drug needs to be taken regularly on seven consecutive days to start demonstrating an effect and that disciplined self-medication needs to continue for six months if a relapse is to be avoided.

Activity 6.1 Reflection

Pause to consider to what extent you have considered motivation when you have been helping patients. Did you ascertain what seemed to sustain patient motivation and did you then use that to adjust how you worked with them?

An outline answer is provided at the end of this chapter.

Motivation

Much of the research and theory associated with human motivation has been conducted within the occupational rather than the healthcare setting. Occupational psychologists are interested in what sustains a highly motivated workforce.

For the purpose of this chapter two theories are summarised and both can be applied to healthcare contexts (see Figure 6.1).

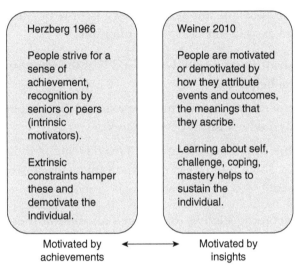

Herzberg 1966	Weiner 2010
People strive for a sense of achievement, recognition by seniors or peers (intrinsic motivators).	People are motivated or demotivated by how they attribute events and outcomes, the meanings that they ascribe.
Extrinsic constraints hamper these and demotivate the individual.	Learning about self, challenge, coping, mastery helps to sustain the individual.

Motivated by achievements ⟷ Motivated by insights

Figure 6.1 Two theories of motivation

The first theory was offered by Herzberg (1966; Alshmemri et al., 2017). Herzberg (1966) argued that we might best understand human motivation in terms of that which rewarded the sense of self, person and achievement, and he called these motivational factors. So, for example, in healthcare, a depressed patient might feel motivated if they could manage without antidepressant medication (the goal). In Herzberg's Two-Factor Theory such intrinsic rewards (that which makes me feel good about myself) are balanced against extrinsic constraints, that which restrains the individual from achieving their ideal state. In depression, constraints might include disruption to sleep, for example, as this leaves patients tired and less able to cope with their negative thoughts.

The second and more complex theory of motivation shared here comes from Weiner (2010). Weiner is less convinced that people are simply motivated by a reward. He argues that human beings habitually attribute meanings to their behaviour and, through this, they develop a richer sense of who they are. People narrate their reality and what represents progress and success there. The more the person understands that narrative, the more motivated and reaffirmed they feel. In this theory it is argued that we attribute meanings to events and to our behaviour.

So, for example, to suffer depression might be explained in terms of predisposing factors – that which made us more prone to the illness. A patient might observe that they always struggle to relate to other people and that this isolates them. Understanding the risks of habitual negative narratives may provide a key to better self-care. Patients can learn to think of themselves as adaptable and increasingly powerful as well.

Whether or not you agree with Weiner probably depends on the extent to which you think human beings are self-analytical. If you think that we constantly evaluate and re-evaluate our actions, then you might be more inclined to find Weiner's theory appealing. What is important about his theory is how our attributions might be characterised. We can explain this using three questions:

1. How stable is that attribution? (Do I explain things the same way all of the time and is the explanation helpful?)

2. How much control do people have in these matters? (It is important to forgive the self if no control could realistically be exercised.)

3. Where it's possible, how much control did I exercise about these events and what does that say about me? (We carry responsibility for our responses to some situations that arise.)

The important observation relating to Weiner's attribution theory is that it offers a potential profile of successful coping. The person who redefines events and their responses in more positive ways is much more likely to go on succeeding and they may be less susceptible to problems in the future. Respecting oneself and one's efforts is critical to endeavour.

Activity 6.2   Critical thinking

Pause now to consider the two competing theories of human motivation and decide what you think might be the implications for helping patients suffering from depression. Do you find one or the other more compelling; if so, why?

An outline answer is provided at the end of this chapter.

Case study: Susan

Last January Susan reached the age of 70. A retired solicitor, she approached her seventh decade with some trepidation. Six years ago she had lost her husband Gregg to lung cancer. As Susan saw it, they were robbed of a retirement together and of the travels that they had put off because of work. Gregg had been in and out of hospital for 14 months receiving palliative treatment. For that period Susan had been her husband's chief carer. Susan didn't remember getting much sleep and sometimes that meant she became irritable with her husband even though she understood just how ill he was.

A few months after Gregg's death, Susan had visited Stewart, her GP, to discuss how low she felt. Susan assumed that this was all to do with grief, but wondered just how long the feelings of despair were meant to continue. Her friends were worried that she had not improved. One friend had suggested bereavement counselling but Susan had insisted that she and Gregg weren't youngsters. Death was part of life and one had to acknowledge that. Still, adaptation seemed to take a long time. Stewart told her that the distinctions between mourning, grief and depression were necessarily vague, but that what she had described was sufficiently concerning that it might be a good idea to complete a six-month course of an antidepressant fluoxetine (Prozac) to help her improve her mood. For it to work, though, she would need to take the medication daily and visit the surgery monthly so that its effect could be monitored.

Her GP explained that Susan also needed to deal with the underlying causes of her low mood. It was important to talk about the loss of her husband and any other negative feelings. To that end, Stewart recommended a course of cognitive behavioural therapy (CBT).

Susan coped reasonably well with her medication and completed the six-month course with few missed tablet days. At the end of the course of medication, however, Susan was anxious to wean herself off her drugs and to find better ways to cope. Despite the GP's advice, she hadn't taken up offers of a talking therapy. Now, aged 70, staring bleakly into the future, Susan felt sure that her illness was back. Susan had given up playing golf and now she stayed up late into the night listening to the news. There were a lot of debates about the economy and Susan had a gloomy feeling that the country was heading towards ruin. Spending a great deal of time worrying about politics, Susan slept poorly. She found it hard to drag herself out of bed in the morning and wondered what there was left to get up for. When you were 70, well, the decades ahead, if you had them at all, were decades of inevitable decline.

After some 'bullying' by an old friend from the golf club, Susan had been persuaded to join a book club. Her friend (Michael) insisted that reading and discussing novels *stopped you maudling*. But Susan simply went through the motions of discussing books, and a mental health nurse, Gillian, who also attended the book club, noticed her emotional flatness. Susan rarely smiled; she was rarely animated. Gillian, who works with a mental health self-help group, was worried that Susan might slip back into acute depression.

Activity 6.3 Speculating

Jot down what you think Susan's problems are and the ways in which these are very personal. What do you think might be problematic if symptoms are relieved but underlying problems are not addressed?

An outline answer is provided at the end of this chapter.

Anticipating patient care

At Susan's request, Gillian agreed to explore her personal problems with Stewart, the GP. This was not a usual referral arrangement, but Susan was distressed by her own lethargy and despair and realised that something new needed to be done. Her GP is a kind man who understood Susan's written request and agreed to meet with Gillian to discuss options for future support. Before they invited Susan to consider possibilities, however, it seemed important to review their potentially differing understanding of depression and its management. Stewart acknowledged Gillian's professional expertise in the field but he was eager to ensure that support measures were practicable and affordable as well.

Salmon (2017), reporting OECD (Organisation for Economic Co-operation and Development) statistics, observes that the UK ranks joint seventh in the world for the incidence of depression. While there are growing numbers of statistics relating to the high incidence of the problem, explanations of how depression arises and what distinguishes it from other conditions are much less clear. Gillian explained, for instance, that patients frequently report a mix of symptoms relating to depression and anxiety. NICE (2009) argues that depression can be diagnosed when symptoms have been present for at least two weeks and affect the individual most days during that period. NICE observes, however, that a full patient history is needed, setting the arrival of problems in a life context.

What was clear, however, and apparent to both Stewart and Gillian, was that depression represents a significant burden on lay carers (people like Michael) (Skundberg-Kletthagen et al., 2014). The persistent nature of depression symptoms and periodic crises in patients means that lay carers suffer a loss of control over their own lives. Lay carers reported living on the patient's terms. Depression increased the chances that the relationship between the patient and their supporters became ambivalent. Lay carers became suspicious of the patient's illness and pessimistic as to whether it could improve. Lay carers struggled to fulfil their own social roles as well as to act as a carer. Any lay carer that contributed to Susan's support might face a considerable burden.

Gillian told Stewart about the experience of depression as reported within focus-group discussions (Frank et al., 2007). While group discussions might help with a variety of things, it was often feelings of irritability with self (my coping) that were relieved. Patients frequently judged themselves and their response to depression and irritability increased their despair. In a rare study exploring patient perceptions of why depression arose and why it persisted, Kelly et al. (2011) proposed that strained interpersonal relationships featured in the experience of illness. Patients who became lonely, who felt alienated from others and isolated, struggled more to deal with their negative emotions. It was debatable whether the strained social relationships occasioned depression or whether they resulted from it (a chicken-and-egg conundrum), but this study did seem to confirm that the way we attribute meanings to our way of living is important in shaping the experience of illness over time.

Stewart said that some of his patients seemed tangled in their problem. Medication alone was rarely a solution even if it did in the interim benefit the chemistry of the brain.

Gillian wasn't surprised that Susan was starting to run into difficulties again. Patients with depression rather easily slipped beneath the radar of the caring services and, as a result, they tended to return to acute-care facilities again and again. Susan had only partly engaged with treatment. While the course of fluoxetine had lifted her mood pro tem, it had not addressed her underlying problems. Goldman et al. (2016) observe that only some 25 per cent of patients complete a coherent treatment package. This was often because the patient accepts some elements of treatment and abandons others. NICE (2009) advocate combination modalities of treatment, often a medication such as fluoxetine and a talking therapy such as CBT. While the medication works neurologically to lift the mood of the patient, the talking therapy operates to help the patient adjust their perceptions of circumstances.

NICE (2009) guidelines advocate a stepped approach to care with medication reserved for well-established and moderate to severe depression. In step one, interventions advocated are psycho-educational in nature (for example, a self-help group) and include regular monitoring. But the problem with this approach is that a healthcare professional might not define the patient's problem as established depression. In this case study, Stewart saw the problem as one of grief and hoped that a course of antidepressant medication might help carry the patient through the transition. He acknowledged, though, that he had not followed up on the package by encouraging Susan to start CBT. Now it had been six years since Susan's husband died.

Practice tip

In some practice areas research evidence is fractured and unclear about the nature of an illness and best treatment options. In such circumstances metanalysis literature reviews can sometimes help you take stock about the quality of evidence available. Manifestly, some form of therapy still has to proceed, so it is then a good idea to alert colleagues to what the literature review offers.

Gillian observed that patients were not always entirely honest with clinicians and that in any case it was difficult to press a solution if the patient believed that taking a pill might prove enough. But she commended talking therapies as important and especially one that had some success amongst patients that she supported. The Talking Sense (2018) initiative describes depression as an emotional problem complicated by interpersonal processes. Patients are often self-critical and they may have actively subverted efforts to help them.

One of the problems with commending a stepped approach to care for Susan was that there were conflicting arguments about whether the approach was viable. Pols et al. (2017), reporting on their own study with Danish patients suffering depression, admitted that the results were mixed. The stepped approach often involved protracted periods of time persevering with a less intrusive form of therapy (at least three months) and that this meant that sometimes a problem might not be adequately addressed for a year or more. Against this, other studies (Van Veer-Tazelaar et al., 2009; Dozeman et al., 2012; Van der Aa et al., 2015) all reported relatively good results. There were three things that were critical to the success of the stepped approach:

1. adequate, well-coordinated talking therapy resources;
2. a systematic approach to assessment and early-stage guidance of the patient (the same case worker, for example);
3. clear conviction about the merits of talking therapies.

Stewart admitted to some ambivalence about counselling. He often found the problem of depression intractable, with the GP's responses being to make do and mend. There was always the gnawing doubt that measures wouldn't work and yet a patient expectation that treatment would achieve quick results. Stewart had read most about CBT. In this treatment patients are helped to understand how their way of reasoning creates behaviours that might trap them within a current problem. The therapist then works with the patient through a series of exercises (new behaviours) that can confirm to the patient that they are capable of living differently (Conklin and Strunk, 2015). The number of sessions that a patient needed to secure progress might be determined by the extent to which patients engaged with activity homework set between times. Such a talking therapy approach might work for Susan, if she could commit to the homework activities.

Against that, however, it also seemed important to Gillian to think about the psycho-social elements of depression as well. Susan had withdrawn from the golf club. It was important to understand why she had given up this source of support, especially when her friend Michael came from that background. Susan didn't have any remaining close friends and, as depression was taxing on others, it seemed a promising idea to re-engage Susan with the golf club, where a wider group of people might help to sustain her morale.

Relating and person-centred care (assessing)

Gillian and Stewart agreed that they assessed depression in different ways, but the solution selection was something that depended largely upon what Susan might feel able to commit to. They felt that three recommendations should be discussed with Susan.

1. First, that she be invited to join Gillian's support group, for which there was no charge. The group engaged in a range of activities designed to start people thinking about the wider world and which enabled them to secure mutual support. Activities included visits to the cinema, TV show reviews, nature walks, visits to art galleries and similar.

2. That Susan be advised to recommence antidepressant medication. Gillian wasn't prepared to involve Susan in the group work until this matter had been agreed. If she was to work with Stewart, to help Susan, then explicit agreement between the three of them had to be secured.

3. That Susan would also be invited to choose a talking therapy, either CBT (that Stewart knew more about) or CfD, which Gillian was familiar with (see below). Irrespective of what Stewart and Gillian speculated might work best, the key issue was: what did Susan feel motivated to work with?

Activity 6.4   Speculating

Gillian is setting in train three elements of support. There is a renewed medication designed to help lift Susan's mood. There is a support group to assure Susan that she is not alone in dealing with her problems. There will then be a carefully chosen talking therapy that helps Susan to reason in a new way about her situation. How do you think the combination of three supports might work to enable Susan to feel that her care is appropriately person-centred?

An outline answer is provided at the end of this chapter.

Hearing the patient narrative

Before exploring the above options, however, Gillian and Stewart agreed to meet with Susan to update their understanding of problems and needs. Both had received a part account of the problem and now it was important to hear the narrative together. A patient's perceptions of their circumstances can change over time. If care was to be adequately coordinated, then it was important that both professionals heard the account together. This would require the allocation of at least one hour's consultation time. Traditional short GP consultation times would be unequal to requirements.

What was important was that Gillian and Stewart understood Susan's assessment of the situation and what might then seem a sustainable and hopeful solution. Hearing the narrative centred upon understanding both need and motivation. Whilst this seemed an unusual amount of time to allocate to one patient in this setting, Gillian assured Stewart that it could be a good investment. Future care requirements might later be reduced and Susan might avoid costly admission to hospital at a later date.

Susan expressed gratitude that both professionals met with her to review the problem. Gillian, though, reminded her that the meeting was a pivotal moment for her as well. If she was to succeed in countering the depression, then she must assess just what her needs were and what support measures she could commit to. The purpose of the meeting was to affirm interest in her situation but also to agree a package of work ahead, that which Susan would be asked to engage in too. Gillian argued that it wasn't entirely useful to talk in terms of treatments; it was better to conceive of the future in terms of work to be done. Simply relying on medication would probably be insufficient.

As Susan narrated her problem, Gillian periodically asked her to pause and summarise a need and the work that might be needed to address that. Stewart jotted down notes, listening intently to how Gillian facilitated the review. Afterwards, Stewart read back to Susan what he had understood as regards her felt needs and future work requirements. These are summarised in Table 6.1.

Table 6.1 Susan's perceived needs and future work implications

Susan's expressed need	Work implication
Finding something to feel hopeful about, a new purpose in living.	The sudden loss of caring/partnering and work responsibilities poses significant challenge to motivation, which has to become more internally referenced. Both group work and a talking therapy might facilitate the exploration and the countering of this.
Searching for a belief in activities, that they might inform, entertain or reassure me.	Susan (and other depressed patients) reports a significant loss of pleasure in activities, including perhaps those eagerly anticipated before. To rediscover pleasure and purpose, though, mood needs to be enhanced (facilitating hope). Onto this can be built activities shared with others that become intrinsically pleasurable and rewarding over time.
Believing that I am valuable, worthy of companionship.	Susan reported low self-esteem. Group work can be valuable in showing that others have felt this too, and that improvements are possible within a supportive environment.
Building a better structure to my day. Retirement and bereavement robbed Susan of roles she had thought important.	Susan admitted 'staring into space' for long periods and then feeling guilty for wasting time. She considered herself intelligent but now 'slothful' and despised herself for that. A talking therapy was important to countering such self-contempt.

Susan's expressed need	Work implication
Resisting the idea that I am fated to develop cancer too (there is no familial history of it being a common problem).	Neither Stewart nor Gillian had previously identified this anxiety, but this too would require countering as part of a talking therapy.
Liking myself through what I do.	Both group work and a talking therapy have the potential to improve self-esteem, through carefully deployed positive feedback.

Activity 6.5   Reflection

Look now again at Table 6.1. Do you think that this very work-orientated, purposeful focus on needs and implications is possible without careful scrutiny of Susan's narrative? What do you think Stewart might have gained from the experience of conducting the interview alongside Gillian? What do you think the implications are for person-centred care, at least where the patient faces a potentially lifelong challenge?

An outline answer is given at the end of this chapter.

Negotiating person-centred care (planning)

Gillian invited Stewart to summarise to Susan the care recommendations that they had previously discussed. This was an important approach because she wished Stewart to feel that Susan remained his patient and because she wanted him to feel that he could invite Susan back to a treatment plan that had previously been only partially adopted by his patient. Gillian explained that she saw this moment as one of building a new beginning. Susan's invitation to Gillian to join the care planning was not meant to be a reproach of Stewart's past recommendations. Instead, it was conceived now as a further insight review of how support might be reconceived. Importantly, too, Gillian explained that she wanted Susan to realise that any commitment made to future plans was directed to both healthcare professionals. There should be no confusion, with Susan making different commitments to each in turn.

Stewart explained that Gillian and he had reviewed current understanding of depression and useful responses and now, with Susan's narrative available, it was time for all three of them to review the options available. It was important to check the fit of such options against the needs that Susan herself had identified. Gillian said that they were collectively examining Susan's problem rather than a textbook depression.

They started with the recommended recommencement of Susan's past medication, something that had indeed lifted her mood and which had been well tolerated before.

Medication, though, would be time limited and incrementally reduced as other measures started to have a beneficial effect. Gillian explained,

> *The medication provides a hope window; it helps you think about possibilities ahead and it's valuable as we build confidence through other help. We want to help you feel receptive to the possibilities.*

Susan cautiously agreed to the measure, once Stewart confirmed that he would not ask her to treat it as a long-term prop for her problems. Susan said that medicine had relied on antidepressants for too long. Gillian interjected that patients and clinicians had alike depended too heavily on just one form of therapy. Stewart seemed relieved that Gillian had countered what had felt like a largely unfair criticism. He resisted the temptation to remind Susan that he had previously recommended CBT.

Gillian described the merits of the support group to Susan, and she in turn asked why that was potentially better than the book club she had attended. Stewart smiled; Susan was an inquisitorial partner in the care planning process. Gillian said,

> *The book club analyses everything, it picks apart the plot of a book, the characterisation and style of the work. Perhaps you need a wider mix of pleasurable shared activities, something not so relentlessly analytical?*

Susan nodded; perhaps so, she agreed.

> *Professional work is relentlessly analytical,* Gillian said, *it becomes something that we are good at and value ourselves by. But if the subject of that becomes yourself, if all there is becomes analysis and judgement, then maybe there is less joy. Retirement can simply be for doing silly, pleasurable things.*
>
> *I wanted to do those with Gregg,* said Susan.
>
> *Yes,* said Gillian, *but there may be others who desire your company too.*

Susan agreed to join the group and to commit to it for four months, sufficient time to assess whether it seemed valuable.

Stewart then introduced the talking therapy options. He described CBT and Gillian summarised CfD. Together they emphasised that this was not a matter of their individual preferences; it was a matter of choosing a therapy that seemed to best inspire confidence in Susan. Susan's choice should reflect her own feelings. She did not have to feel she was favouring either Stewart or Gillian's personal recommendation.

Gillian explained that whilst CBT focused upon learning new behaviours, in CfD there was a stronger emphasis on the emotional component of depression. Patients were encouraged to narrate their experiences in rather more depth, much as Susan had just done to identify her first needs (Haake, 2017). Whilst many people imagined that psychological counselling required long periods of time in therapy, CfD was typically scheduled as a series of 8–12 sessions, comparable in commitment to CBT. The therapist did not prescribe measures to the patient but instead facilitated a personal enquiry into how something psychological had meant that the patient had become stuck in their response to life. CfD was designed to help the patient select their own future way forward, something that Gillian believed might be additionally advanced both by antidepression medication and by a support group.

Susan worried that the counselling could become unduly intrusive, unpicking her relationship with Gregg, for instance. But Gillian explained that irrespective of whether CBT or CfD was used, there would be a need to identify problems. Therapists from both traditions were respectful of the work done by the patient as they reflected on their circumstances. There was no judgement about what good living must consist of, but patients still had to understand what stopped them from engaging in activities that seemed personally desirable. The therapist would:

- help Susan identify what seemed to block her from advancing new plans;
- help her to understand how memories fuelled personal assessment of circumstances today and plans for the future;
- help her appraise her habitual ways of responding to change. In this regard both CBT and CfD were action orientated, helping the patient to plan new ways of acting in the future.

Gillian said that CBT perhaps emphasised exercises and homework rather more, whilst CfD emphasised a quiet introspection on emotions and beliefs, but neither therapy dictated what the patient *must* do. Therapy of both kinds was facilitative rather than directive.

Susan said that she was prepared to commit to an initial course of up to 12 sessions of CfD but she wished to reserve the right to withdraw if the programme did not seem to help. Stewart said that he wouldn't recommend mixing and matching, or suddenly switching therapies; whatever Susan elected to use, she had to give it a fair chance to succeed. Gillian agreed. As she explained, *We are talking work here, Susan, not treatment.* The therapies of both kinds required commitment on her part as well. For that reason, a minimum of at least eight sessions should be completed, working with a therapist that Gillian would introduce her to, before any withdrawal.

Practice tip

Clinicians have to have confidence in recommended treatments or therapies, so it is valuable periodically to rehearse their merits in conversation. You might be confronted with other proposals, including alternative medicine ones. It is entirely reasonable to admit that you don't know about all options but that you're willing to research more. Nonetheless, if you still have doubts, share those honestly before a plan is agreed.

> ## Activity 6.6   Critical thinking
>
> Stewart and Gillian characterised talking therapy options and Susan made her choice. She felt able to raise questions and concerns. How important do you think it is in this instance to characterise therapy as a form of work versus treatment? In your experience, how accustomed are patients to making an active contribution to therapies?
>
> *An outline answer is provided at the end of this chapter.*

Collaborating on person-centred care (implementing)

Before summarising the collaborative patient care, it is worth pausing for a moment to understand what is involved in the above plan. Susan became engaged in three different kinds of meetings on a regular basis. First, she met with Stewart to recommence her medication and then checked in with him monthly by video link to discuss how the treatment was working. Stewart was keen to understand how the social support group and a talking therapy were also influencing Susan's progress. Stewart described this as a personal discovery as well. He knew relatively little about CfD and had only recently become engaged in social support prescription, referring patients to services that worked in very different ways to medicine (Mercer, 2018). He wished to understand how Susan thought about her support with three different kinds of help. Did they (as he put it) 'orchestrate in her head'? If they did, then he wished to describe the potential benefits and responsibilities of the same for other future patients that might be referred.

Susan's second set of meetings were with the support group that Gillian facilitated. These were weekly events where up to a dozen individuals met, although group members were encouraged to stay in touch in the interim through a Facebook messaging arrangement. Susan described the group as 'less intense' than the book club, where many of the members had been aspiring authors. The group included a wider variety of members, all of whom had faced a health or personal difficulty, but all of whom made a weekly commitment to learning something new. At the first meeting that Susan attended there was a show-and-tell evening where two of the members related their struggles in mastering a skill (making sourdough bread and learning the geography of a town before the individual became a taxi driver). Such sessions Gillian described not only as ice-breakers, but as resource insights; fellow group members had skills and experiences to share. Susan was pleasantly surprised and had been persuaded to plan a future talk of her own, 'Nightmares and dream moves – a description of house conveyancing'.

The last set of (weekly) meetings were with Bruce, her counsellor. These had taken a little longer to book and were conducted one to one in a quiet and comfortable sitting-room environment. Susan described these as the hard-work sessions, but conceded that as her medication had started to take beneficial effect, she felt more equal to the sessions than she had anticipated. Gillian asked her how they seemed to be going but emphasised that Susan was at liberty to share as much or as little as she chose. Bruce had encouraged her to tell him stories from her recent life, the time of depression and before. He promised that whatever she thought of as important counted as valuable to him. He asked brief questions to clarify points, but did not interrupt with recommendations. Susan analogised the sessions as 'a look through my garden'. Bruce might draw her attention to particular plants, but without prescribing what each meant or what she should do about such matters. At the next session Susan was at liberty to pick up on threads, exploring what she had already thought about, determining whether something still seemed the same way, or whether she now wished to think about it differently.

I was struck by the parallel nature of the work and by the relatively light-touch monitoring of progress as support developed. Gillian became the touchstone 'how are things going?' reference point because she seemed so receptive. But the coordination was much less structured, rather less regulated, than we might expect in an institutional setting. The sense-making work, the 'mixing and mood work', as Susan described it, was left to herself. Each of the therapists or groups offered a resource, but did not directly attempt to dictate improvements in her daily life.

I want to illustrate this eclectic, extremely person-centred focus of collaborative work with reference to insights that Susan gained into why she had not returned to the golf club, a place of potential support after her husband died. Through 'storying' for Bruce, Susan realised that she had become angry about the golf club and how it seemed to function. Gregg had been a successful golfer with a low handicap, whilst she described herself as a social golfer. Bruce had asked whether that was like Après ski and she explained it was more than that. Yes, many of the lady golfers enjoyed drinks at the bar, but there was a different mindset. Amongst the stronger golfers there was a fierce competitiveness that seemed to translate as disdain for those less competitively orientated. In consequence the golf club had become defined by two camps. Susan had felt angry about this and angry at Gregg for not acknowledging the divide that she felt existed there. Bruce asked whether the serious golfers' opinion mattered a great deal to her and she had admitted that, before, it had. She wanted their approval. Now, she was less sure. If she did decide to return, she might even take up a social membership, refusing to play 'mental games on the green'.

Gillian reported this theme to me and explained how Susan had then independently transferred the debate to the social support group. How much did winning matter? How important was it to be the best at something? She obtained an array of opinions including one gambler who ruefully observed that beating the odds could become a dangerous obsession. Questing to become an expert gambler could mean falling into greater debt. Gillian had later asked her what she made of that. Susan replied that things could be worth doing simply for the distraction of it. Life could be about more than performance.

This interlude seems almost whimsical, doesn't it? But I suspect that it demonstrates something important about person-centred care in collaboration. This is that the direction of work, the discoveries of work, are personally referenced. The discoveries are about what makes sense to the patient, about what in this context lifts mood and engenders confidence. We cannot readily identify which 'input' had the most profound effect on Susan's morale, but it seems likely that the biggest impact was when they were mixed together by her. So Bruce facilitated the opportunity to stop and think about her assumptions, about an anger she had not previously articulated. But the normality of debating success, what really mattered, was then built in the social support group. The readiness to persevere with storying, reflecting, may in the first instance have been strongly aided by her medication.

Susan incrementally adopted the role of enquirer and her different therapists adopted the roles of supporters and facilitators. This is in sharp contrast to many other acute-care therapeutic settings, where the healthcare professional retains a larger leadership role. That the healthcare team did not have absolute certainty of what therapy might achieve demanded of them a considerable degree of trust and patience, allowing Susan to conduct her own enquiries into what hindered a more satisfying way to live after the death of her husband. Periodically, Susan sought reassurance from each of the three professionals assisting her and each provided a cautious review of what seemed to be improving. In each instance the healthcare professionals asked her to consider what work she wanted to attend to next.

Activity 6.7   Reflection

How do the above insights into person-centred care work in action make you feel? What seems to be involved in helping the patient to conduct their own work, to make their own incremental decisions? In mental healthcare this approach is likely to seem more familiar, but what about within adult nursing, child health or learning disability care? Choosing to work in a person-centred care way may have profound implications for what you do or say.

An outline answer is given at the end of this chapter.

Evaluating person-centred care (evaluating)

After the first month of the three therapies that Susan was using, Gillian proposed that she meet again with Stewart and herself to discuss progress to date. Bruce, her CfD therapist, was unavailable to join the meeting but he asked to receive a summary of any insights shared. Gillian explained to me that the timing of the meeting was important. A month into the new package of agreed care, there was the prospect that medication would show a beneficial effect. At this point too, Susan would have completed four group events and three counselling sessions with Bruce. The meeting would provide insights well ahead of a cut-off point where Susan might theoretically withdraw from one or more of the therapies. Gillian explained too that it was important with regard to motivation theory. At this point in time Susan would likely understand what narrating illness and response entailed; what it meant to work for control over mood and daily living once more.

Stewart described the meeting to Susan as a 'discoveries session', one where she might take stock of work to date. It was not assumed that progress would be made. Indeed, it was possible that a patient might recount a growing series of problems and fears. He had treated other patients who had received CBT where the problem had initially seemed larger. Attending to a difficulty, articulating it in some way, could make it seem more daunting still. Nonetheless, it seemed important now to help Susan evaluate events so far and to possibly request any necessary further guidance or assistance.

Susan welcomed the meeting, although she did admit to some anxiety regarding it. When you completed staff appraisals, the employee was always asked to appraise their own work first before a manager then commented on performance. The therapy had been described as work so it was easy to see stock taking as an appraisal of performance. Gillian nodded, yes, the parallel seemed compelling. However, she observed that any judgement made would be her own; it was Susan who would report satisfaction or dissatisfaction. Susan was setting her own path, establishing a happier and more purposeful daily form of living.

What have you discovered so far? Gillian asked her after coffee had been served.

Susan surprised Gillian and Stewart with her account. She took out a notebook which she had kept to aid her discussions with Bruce. Methodically, she summarised the discoveries (see Table 6.2).

Table 6.2 Susan's discoveries

Discoveries	Notes
Many of my difficult feelings centre on retirement, not specifically on the loss of my husband.	Stewart asked what Susan thought retired life would seem like and she imagined that it would seem leisurely and a relief. But that was more enjoyable with a partner, and he was now gone. Nonetheless, retirement involved assigning meaning to your day, motivating yourself more than you anticipated. It was work of a different kind.

(Continued)

Table 6.2 (Continued)

Discoveries	Notes
I have been ill-prepared for retirement, imagining that daily activities would be readily filled and that they would have intrinsic pleasure and meaning.	Gillian reflected that activities could seem more precious when time was limited, when you couldn't access them so readily. Motivation was undermined, perhaps, if you could do them at any time.
Being 70 involves work of its own; I am too young and healthy to feel infirm and yet there are limits to my energy.	Stewart asked, 'when are we old?' and Susan grinned and said, 'you are old ten years more than now!' So old age was relative, and waiting for possible infirmity, a cancer, was a counsel of despair.
I have shut out old friends from the golf course, partly because I feared pity and partly because of anger about divisions that I recognised there.	Gillian asked whether the fear of pity was realistic, given what she knew of selected friends. Susan answered no, friends had genuinely wanted to help her. They wanted her company. It wasn't a memorial kindness towards Gregg. Susan had applied for a social membership at the golf club. 'You might play again?' Stewart ventured, to which Susan replied, 'a step at a time'.
People from many walks of life are lovely and have something to share, something to teach me. I don't have to worry how I seem to them, whether I sound professional in some regard.	Gillian asked what the support group prompted in her. Susan said, 'laughter – life is a little bit ridiculous and we are too serious too soon'.

I agreed with Gillian that this summary signalled a significant uplift in Susan's mood and a renewed sense of purpose. She had begun to hope for better days in the future and moreover believed that she could start to change her mood through her own activities. *Susan has found agency,* Gillian explained; *she believes that she makes her life better.* For now, though, the medication support was important, enhancing feelings of progress and personal value. It would take a series of successes, in therapy, through the social group support, before she could be confident of carrying on, regardless of adversity that might lie ahead. Gillian explored with Susan what she might now like to bring to the social support group herself and what help they might offer as she ventured back to the golf club. It was important, Gillian explained, to consider next issues as well as to celebrate that already learned or achieved.

Bruce was pleased with the progress report and especially with Susan's ability to summarise issues so succinctly and clearly. It suggested to him that she had distilled lessons secured through storying and that these were reasonably clear. As he explained, we search for footholds before reaching for something more. That Susan was testing out explanations and ideas in the support group was another positive sign. *She's not always earnest about that either,* explained Gillian; *sometimes she laughs at her own concerns. She is starting to see worries in proportion.*

Over the coming weeks either Gillian or Bruce invited Susan to take stock again of her progress. The stock taking happened every three weeks. Susan passed the points where she said she would determine whether the therapies worked. She proceeded on without comment; the work had become intrinsic to her passing weeks. At the end of the 12 weeks of CfD Susan, Stewart and Gillian met again to sum up what the plan had achieved. On this occasion Susan evaluated the service received and what this had meant to her. She made the following points:

- recovering didn't seem possible without the medication priming. It had felt a reassurance, something chemical to help sustain psychological work;
- the support group had been joyful, unjudgemental and reaffirming. She hoped to continue in the group if that was possible for another month or two until golf friendships and activities were re-established;
- the counselling had seemed taxing but Bruce was entirely calm and implacably confident that 'something good was possible'. Susan was unsure whether that was due to his techniques or personality; she only knew that it worked.

The group agreed then that Susan's medication would be tapered off over the next four months and that the support group was a good means to monitor how Susan felt about that transition and coping more herself. The CfD sessions concluded at this juncture and Stewart wrote to Bruce to congratulate him on the contribution made in this case. Gillian asked Stewart whether he had enjoyed the team working in support of Susan. Stewart affirmed that he had. It had been pleasant, encouraging and yes, it was empowering when he had previously felt embattled helping people with anxiety and depression.

Person-centred care insights

I think that this case study offers a number of encouragements for nurses exploring person-centred care. The first and perhaps most major of these relates to motivation and the possible role of storying or narrating experience of illness and recovery. At the start of this chapter I laid special emphasis upon motivation and offered two theories of how this might work. Weiner's (2010) theory of motivation sustained by insights and attributions seems supported in this case study. Susan's work was to narrate the way in which she thought about her circumstances and what seemed possible in the future. Where such narration focuses first upon blocks to more positive thinking, then seizing of opportunities, as it does in CfD, there is an opening for the patient to better understand how their feelings and reasoning shape progress.

The focus on feelings, mood and motivation means that this is quintessentially a personal rather than simply a medical problem. Unless the personal problem is addressed, the medical problems of depression might return and accelerate away. Hospital care, long-term medication and perhaps crisis management thereafter may represent a very significant cost to healthcare services as well as a threat to the wellbeing of the patient.

In healthcare, nurses often don't feel that they have the time to attend in depth to patient perceptions and feelings, yet this case study illustrates what an important and major contribution care in this area can be. That which is personal, that which the patient perceives and then conceives in terms of what represents a problem, needs sometimes, as here, to steer the plan of care.

Narrative analysis is used in person-centred care to better understand the patient, their perceptions and needs, but it seems evident in this case study that patient narrating can have a therapeutic as well as a logistical purpose too. To narrate is to learn – to map difficulties and perhaps then to identify routes towards a healthier life ahead. The more the patient understands how their reasoning might trap them in current difficulties, the more they can realise that they have power to determine future courses of action. This realisation, that perceptions and habitual forms of reasoning can imprison people, is important. It focuses attention on what the therapeutic work of the patient might centre upon. In this case study Susan was acquainted with the need for such work. Her outcome would be as much determined by her own learning and decision making as by medication or therapies provided by Gillian and her colleagues. In this instance Susan was ready to respond to that challenge. She had spent six years trying to make sense of the loss of her husband and discovered that medication alone was not equal to the challenge posed by depression. If she was to make a more contented life, then she would have to learn from her experience and embrace new opportunities afforded her by healthcare staff members.

The case study neatly illustrates how patients can determine the plan of action and shape what is done to address a healthcare problem. In this instance there were a range of possible therapies that might have helped Susan, although Stewart and Gillian recommended two that they were more confident about. One of the roles of the person-centred care nurse in such circumstances is to help narrow down options, to set forth alternatives so that the patient can assess that which might have a better fit to personal circumstances and needs. In this case study Susan was understandably cautious. She wanted to manage the risk of intrusion that she associated with counselling and she reserved the right to opt out of therapy provided that she had given it reasonable time to assist her. Susan understood, though, that partnering Gillian and Stewart in the plan of care required personal commitment as well. It was unrealistic to conceive of herself as a passive consumer to whom therapy was applied.

What I think may seem surprising, however, is the relatively looser coordination and care plan work, and the acceptance that Susan would marshal her own relationship work with the GP, the support group and the counsellor. This can seem rather 'try it and see', with evolving goals and with much less supervision than we might associate with, for instance, a group rehabilitation programme. Accepting that the patient becomes the investigator means accepting that we become facilitators and supporters. We cannot do the transitional work for the patient. We can encourage, console, reassure, but we cannot direct in these particular circumstances. There seems then a pivotal point that operates around the negotiation-of-care stage. If the patient is to become a manager, an enquirer or investigator, then that shapes the roles that nurses and others can offer. This requires trust. In this instance it meant judging that Susan was ready to make a new beginning and to counter her depression in a more coherent way. Sometimes, nurses and doctors might have to realise that it is better to let go a little, to commend or direct rather less. Sometimes it may be necessary to accept that the final outcome may be different than we expected, but still potentially beneficial in the patient's own terms.

The final insight that I would share with you on this case is that person-centred care has the potential to improve interdisciplinary working in healthcare. Provided that stakeholders feel able to commit to helping the patient in more imaginative ways, there is the potential to make beneficial professional discoveries along the way. Notice at the outset how Gillian met with Stewart first to ascertain their different perspectives on depression and treatment. This seemed important when much depression care remains in flux, and debates continue about what works best. Had these colleagues not explored their experience and views at the outset, disputes about best therapy or case management could have arisen later. Notice Gillian's wisdom as she recognises how Stewart might have felt about her own intervention when Susan had previously not followed his medical prescription. It required wisdom on Gillian's part to manage professional territory. What enabled her to do this was the realisation that person-centred care was a legitimate interest and goal of different healthcare professionals. The outcome of this case study was entirely positive. Susan eventually stopped taking medication and was able to manage her periodic dark days by understanding the propensity to think in more negative terms. She understood how a habitual narration could stymy life opportunities. That she was able to do this seemed in no small part due to the successful collaboration and trust between Gillian, Stewart and Bruce, her counsellor.

Chapter summary

Person-centred care has potential in helping patients with what can seem intractable problems. It does so because it acknowledges the pivotal role of the patient. Within person-centred care there is sometimes scope for the patient to become the investigator, the critical appraiser of what has been discovered and what now might be mastered. This seems a very long way from the more limited partnership possibilities that you read about in Chapter 3, those pertaining in some acute-care contexts. At issue perhaps, then, is who bears the perceived cost and benefits of decisions? If the patient is confronted with daily difficulties when no change is contemplated, then they may become extremely motivated and that has the potential to change the role that a nurse might fulfil. In some acute care the costs and benefits of decisions are described by clinicians, and sometimes projected as arising months or years in the future. The psychology of motivation operates a little differently.

(Continued)

(Continued)

In chronic health contexts there has been much more time for the patient to become acquainted with what treatment can and cannot do. In this case study Susan was ready to respond to offers of assistance and to persevere with work that attended to that.

This case study, like its three predecessors, highlights the importance of several recurring themes. The first is the importance of discovering and working with patient narratives. If narratives are not uncovered, if they are not worked with, then collaboration might falter. Healthcare operates instead with more abstract issues, not that which is experienced, perceived and felt, and recommendations might seem less valid or urgent. The second theme concerns that of roles. Nurses and patients alike play roles and the better these are understood and embraced, the greater the potential for the advancement of mutually agreed goals. Roles, however, need to be learned and sometimes reviewed or augmented. In this case study, Stewart the GP commenced his own journey of discovery, exploring a new solution to a recurring problem in his practice. The third theme is that of collaboration. What collaboration focuses upon may vary widely. In some situations, the medical problem dominates; in others, the personal problem comes more to the fore and that may become the lens to solving underlying medical problems. Sometimes how we think determines what we can achieve.

Activities: Brief outline answers

Activity 6.1 Reflection (p130)

I have tended to scrutinise motivation when the patient's progress has faltered. I have tended to use motivation insights as a rescue response, especially when I used to help patients to live with disfigurement.

But I now think that understanding motivation is pivotal to person-centred care. When you ask a patient what motivates them, you signal an interest in what matters most to them. Understanding and using motivation theory is part of the person-centred-care counter to trite prescription. Instead of saying that you have illness X and the response here is therapy Y, you acknowledge that therapies are tools for patients and that requires motivation.

Motivation remains important in both acute care and in later stages of care where the personal problem might be more apparent. In acute care we need to consider to what extent the patient is motivated to accept what we believe to be necessary treatment. That means we must understand how the patient perceives risk. In later care we must consider motivation in the context of understanding what sustains the patient in what sometimes becomes a radically altered lifestyle. Managing chronic illness can seem exhausting so we had better have regard for motivation.

Activity 6.2 Critical thinking (p132)

One of the positives of Herzberg's (1966) theory of motivation is that it highlights reasoning that patients are likely to find relatively easy to understand. One of the problems, though, is that many patients' circumstances are more complex. Someone suffering from a chronic illness, such as depression, has to identify repeated rewards for themselves, and the fact that these perhaps aren't sustainable limits the utility of this theory.

My personal preference then is to think of motivation as a more dynamic process, one which we fuel through recurring new accounts of what we are working at (Weiner, 2010). Many of the mental healthcare talking therapies rely on this emphasis of attribution, adding new meaning to what we have committed to. In mental healthcare there is a strong focus upon understanding narratives and then using the same to redefine ourselves. If attribution theory of this kind appeals to you, then you may already see life in project terms. If you prefer an effort-and-rewards understanding of motivation, then you might see life in less strategic terms. Life seems happier with a greater degree of happenchance.

Activity 6.3 Speculating (p134)

I believe that Susan faces a depression that might once have been described as reactive but which now risks becoming chronic. It is six years since her husband died, and right now she anticipates life in her 70s with a sense of foreboding. We might reasonably speculate that Susan is unsure now how to reclaim a happiness that she anticipated characterising retirement for many years to come.

Susan nursed her husband whilst he was ill, so she is keenly aware of what illness can do to the quality of life for an older person. Notice how a well-meaning friend has had to cajole her to take part in a book club. This may produce feelings of ambivalence for someone in Susan's situation. Why must I be jollied along?

One of the things that nurses can find hard to do is to appreciate the extent and depth of despair that depressed patients sometimes feel. We might worry that mapping of the same will only deepen the patient's sense of futility. Yet without understanding the patient's perceptions, it becomes very hard to support a recovery. Susan needs assistance to address her emotions; the sense of loss, anger or confusion. If symptoms are merely suppressed, then they may return, perhaps explosively, at a later date. Arguably all human beings carry some emotional baggage, doubts and worries about earlier life, but for patients who are clinically depressed this can become all-enveloping. It is for this reason that some form of talking therapy needs to be combined with medication.

Activity 6.4 Speculating (p137)

One of the challenges in many mental healthcare situations is that the patient starts from the midst of the problem. They have to make sense of their distress. Compare this to a physical healthcare problem, for instance arthritis. There the problem can be localised and objectified. My wrists are painful in the morning, my hips or back are sore because of deterioration in the joints there. In mental health problems, that which is the self seems attacked. It is much harder to examine the problem, the patient sometimes realising that even their thought processes have become alien. Orchestration of support in such circumstances becomes vital.

Medication assists the depressed patient by bolstering neurochemicals such as serotonin that sustain a positive mood for the patient. Whilst clinicians might debate what comes first in depression, a neurochemical change or psycho-social reasoning problems, what seems compelling is the need to affect both together. Susan needs assistance to explore her mental health problem. It requires bravery to examine where the problem originated and how it is now shaping life in a negative way. Talking therapies provide the tools and the challenge necessary to do that. They help the patient to direct their reflection in particular ways. But that challenge in this instance seems better met with additional assistance, from a social support group. The group not only provides hope and solace as the patient perseveres with a therapy, but it might also help someone like Susan realise the rewards of socialising.

Activity 6.5 Reflection (p139)

It probably won't surprise you to learn that I think narrative analysis is vital in person-centred care and especially in a case study such as Susan. We arrive at needs through an account of experiences and what within those seems important to change. The psychological process of narrating involves a transition from noticing things (what happened) to conceptions of what events imply. This event was threatening, that event taught me something, the last event reaffirmed something that I believe (or the contrary). What counts as a need is a realisation that a particular series of events, a collection of changes, now necessitates some kind of change for me. I have to think, act, feel, behave differently. To arrive at even this seemingly brief table of insights, Susan has completed a lot of psychological work.

In this case study Stewart listened to Gillian's interviewing skills with considerable respect. Afterwards he explained to me that it was obvious Gillian treated every insight as being as tangible as the body signs that he was used to focusing upon. The ability to make each idea real, something communicable, that he then jotted down was a considerable skill that he admired. Gillian had a clear conviction that the narrative mattered and that it represented beliefs and values held by Susan. The narrative wasn't transitory, a passing moment's reflection that wouldn't necessarily be valid in an hour's time. The ability to 'nail down a narrative' in this way gave Susan hope. What she said mattered to Gillian and it could then become part of a package of help. Stewart explained that he realised just how strategic, how valuable, a conversation could be.

I believe that making psychological issues real, accessible and amenable to some form of intervention is at the heart of person-centred care. It rapidly assures the patient of the nurse's respect and their interest in the patient's life experienced. Person-centred care is psychological in nature, something that complements all the psychomotor skills of the nurse, the evidence and knowledge that he or she deploys. It is what enables the patient to feel cared for, as well as treated.

Activity 6.6 Critical thinking (p142)

Much of my clinical work was associated with helping patients to overcome problems of disfigurement. I dealt with patients who had been injured through trauma, and those damaged by cancer or its treatment. Whilst the public might be urged to assess disfigured individuals more respectfully, work remained for patients to manage a range of different reactions that they might encounter in others.

No matter what my skills were in helping patients with altered body image challenges, the psychological adjustment work was their own. In depression too I argue there is benefit in conceiving of rehabilitation as work. In such work the patient sets their own objectives, catalogues progress and reviews resources. Work has good days and bad days. Conceiving of adjustment as work serves to counter self-pity, which patients could become liable to. The notion of treatment is arguably more problematic in such contexts. The treatment might fail. Perhaps it was the wrong treatment; perhaps it was ended too soon or carried on too long? Treatment can be seen as prescribed by experts, and this risks damaging the notion of collaboration that might be so important in psychological care. In much psychological care the patient brings expertise of their own, insights into how they habitually cope and what motivates them most of all. Patients vary markedly in their assumptions about collaborative work with healthcare staff, some assuming that their role is entirely a passive one. In my experience the patients who achieve the most are those that are active collaborators in care.

Activity 6.7 Reflection (p144)

I am sometimes surprised by what hampers a patient from making effective changes. The problems in a person's mind seem much larger than I imagine them to be, given my own life experiences. But this is what a narrative-led, person-centred enquiry sometimes leads to. We discover what counts as a problem for the other person. The size and the complexity of the problem is linked to the personal history of the patient. So we might have to suspend judgement, and attend in detail to what exercises the patient and work with what they present. Whilst we can anticipate a great deal of likely care requirements (and need to), and draw on evidence, we have as well to understand the way in which patients process experience.

Helping patients to conduct their own care work requires that we appreciate the different ways in which they reason. Some of that may seem unusual, less direct than we perhaps might imagine. There is always the pressure of time and finite resources available, but then what is finally achieved was always influenced by what the patient feels able to collaborate upon. We create a dissonance for ourselves if we insist that the patient outcome must include our desired accomplishments whilst the process of getting there remains under the control of the patient. There are probably hundreds of different possible 'satisfactory' patient outcomes associated with an illness such as depression, each outcome judged individually by the patients themselves. Patients fit illness to their own circumstances. They draw on varying amounts of personal psychology and support resource beyond that offered by nurses and other healthcare staff. So we probably should evaluate progress, success, in rather more nuanced terms.

In healthcare fields beyond mental health this more nuanced review of our work might seem rather strange. We are used to working with more clearly defined illness; we have a range of treatments that might be deemed a cure. There is a tendency for us to rely more heavily upon notions of subject expertise, rather than compassionate assistance. In these fields we might feel a more urgent need to 'make things right' for the patient. Certainly, we need to offer sound, evidence-based advice, to counter identified risks, but there remains a case to be made too for creating more space, and assigning more responsibility to the patient, for what the patient chooses and how they solve problems in a life context.

Further reading

Kennerley, H, Kirk, J and Westbrook, D (2017) *An Introduction to Cognitive Behavioural Therapy: Skills and Applications.* 3rd edition. London: SAGE.

The market is awash with self-help textbooks relating to most of the talking therapies, including CBT. But the approach is more complex than such textbooks suggest and the process requires skilled practice. This well-established textbook is a good summary of the stages of therapy and reviews the different theoretical traditions that shape CBT in practice. If you wish to secure an appreciation of what the therapy might offer, this is a valuable resource.

Lewis, G (2016) *Sunbathing in the Rain: A Cheerful Book About Depression.* London: Harper Perennial.

It is possible to write about an illness with both wit and insight. Gwyneth Lewis manages that and then some. As depression is potentially a lifelong illness with recurrence of problems over time, a memoire is well suited to offering patient insights.

Murphy, D (2019) *Person-Centred Experiential Counselling for Depression.* 2nd edition. London: SAGE/BCAP.

Each of the different talking therapies have their advocates and debates still continue as regards what is most effective. This textbook, though, provides a measured review of this counselling approach and its humanistic underpinnings. There is a good summary of how counsellors proceed and what is expected of the client in return. Irrespective of your chosen perspective on talking therapies, this book represents an interesting read as it operates at the juncture of what nurses sometimes mean by person-centred care, psychological support more generally and what counselling adds to our understanding of narrative and narrating.

Useful websites

Depression represents an excellent opportunity to revisit how we narrate the experience of illness. It is also an opportunity to examine how we (as nurses) narrate depression to others. Narrative is at the centre of depression and so are analogies. It is very hard to describe depression without recourse to imagery. That this is necessary, capturing the scale and the extent of a mood locked in on sadness and despair, tells us something about the shortfall of vocabulary and the fear and distrust we anticipate that mental illness occasions.

So I want to encourage you to view three narratives on YouTube (**www.youtube.com**), each about depression. The first is a lengthy account of depression (some 30 minutes long) by a highly articulate and sometimes amusing man called Andrew Solomon (search 'Andrew Solomon: Depression, the secret we share'). It is a talk that he delivered in 2013 but which remains entirely relevant today. Andrew narrates the depth of depression, contrasting it with the adaptive array of emotions that people enjoy in health. He explains the extent to which it can dominate a life. I think it is well worth watching, not only to build empathy for patients but also to speculate about what patients can learn from others who have (as it were) landscaped the condition. See what you think!

Two other worthwhile videos to watch on YouTube are much shorter and represent narratives of depression that professionals share with the public. The first by Helen Farrell (search 'Helen Farrell: What is depression?') represents a very simple but balanced summary of depression, a real medical condition that merits attention, respect and treatment as much as any other. Notice the comparisons made between physical illness and depression. This is conceptualisation and it is something that person-centred care nurses use a lot when helping patients. 'You might think of it this way ...'

The second professional narrative is produced by the World Health Organization (WHO) and makes use of the black dog analogy that Winston Churchill (Britain's World War II leader) often referred to (search 'WHO: I had a black dog, his name was depression'). What is compelling about this narrative is not simply the clever use of cartoon graphics, but also how the authors explain that you can transform depression if you reconceptualise the problems that you face. Talking therapy involves a lot of such reconceptualisation work and I hope that you can see its potential too.

Chapter 7 Checking back and looking forward

Chapter aims

After reading this chapter, you will be able to:

- reflect upon what the case studies of this book have taught you about person-centred care;
- demonstrate awareness of the outstanding challenges and opportunities that lie ahead for person-centred care in the future.

Introduction

In this final chapter of the book I want to help you to take stock of what you have already read so far and to peer briefly into the future. As you read in Chapter 1, person-centred care developed as part of a wider, more liberal healthcare philosophy, one that resonates clearly with values in nursing. We wish to support patients, to help them liberate themselves from the restrictions and threats associated with illness or injury and to live well in terms that are both healthy and personally meaningful (Backman et al., 2019). We hope to help people feel well, something rather more than just being disease- or injury-free. We hope to help patients have better charge of their life circumstances. By any standards, this is an ethical but exacting order to fulfil. As we saw in Chapter 2, it has implications for the way that care is organised and the steps that nurses follow as they build a relationship with the patient. We can only share the negotiation and planning of care if patients feel equal to such work (Byrne et al., 2020). The person-centred care challenge is always in the detail: how do we combine sound evidence, clinical experience, empathy and reflective practice to serve the patient well?

Having read the four case studies within this book, I hope you have realised that person-centred care is not a formula that you can simply apply in every context. Person-centred care involves relationship building and it raises serious questions about the roles that nurses, patients and lay carers might adopt. Person-centred care becomes a care philosophy that demands something of patients, just as it sets out responsibilities for nurses and other healthcare professionals (Price, 2017). Nurses cannot simply make patients engage with them in person-centred care.

However, person-centred care is not only shaped by what patients feel able to engage in; it is also influenced to a significant degree by the environment in which care is delivered. In acute-care, hospital-based environments, contact time between the patient and an individual nurse may be severely limited. The patient encounters a wide range of staff for brief interludes of time and the extent to which the care is person-centred depends much more upon how care systems work. Some healthcare trusts might strive to personalise care, individualising the care planning process, but as a truly bespoke care is difficult to cost, manage and update, it is more likely that care in these settings is conceived of in much more standard care package terms (Mintzberg, 2017). In acute care there is a risk that the patient feels they have been swallowed by a system.

In other settings within the community, for instance those associated with chronic illness and the management of lifestyle change, there is greater scope to personalise care. It is no coincidence that some of the greatest advances in person-centred care have been conceived of within care-of-older-people environments (McCormack, 2021). Here the care relationship is often lengthy, and the nurse has time to get to know the patient well. The divide between that which counts as a medical and a personal problem blurs and the nurse realises that addressing personal problems (those mediated strongly by perceptions and feelings) is often the very best way to address a medical problem as well (e.g. diabetes, confusion).

Medical and personal problems

In the first edition of this book I set person-centred care in rather more political terms: a contest between different care systems and values. I argued that the nurse can feel torn between different philosophies of what should be offered to patients. Some of those problems remain today. Bespoke care is expensive to provide. Serious questions remain to be addressed about what healthcare systems can realistically offer (Ross, 2020). There may be some care options, those that the patient especially desires, that are only available through personal purchase or a health insurance supplementary cost. Nurses have to operate within an economic as well as a philosophical care system.

I think now, though, that the majority of person-centred care challenges are not simply political or cost-related, but about clarifying what the realistic work of the nurse is within acute versus longer-term care relationship settings. If we characterise acute, hospital-based care settings, the care encounter is often comparatively short. Patients spend less time in hospital and those that are there are often more acutely ill. A patient who finds themselves in hospital, perhaps at short notice, and facing the need for significant treatment, is poorly placed to negotiate care in the way that some would wish to see. This is because:

1. The patient often arrives at a psychological disadvantage (e.g. Harrison et al., 2017). They are at once overwhelmed with information and yet short of critically important information as well. A battery of investigations, the incremental nature of the diagnostic process and the debated best-treatment options make it harder for the patient to participate equally in care deliberation. It is not that clinicians are unwilling to explain issues; it is that a high volume of complex information is difficult to comprehend and make personal decisions upon if you are stressed.

2.   Patients are operating outside of their psychological comfort zone, in a setting where healthcare professionals have the majority of power (through expertise and information) and where the patient might be distracted by pain and other worries about what illness or injury means for their lives (e.g. Ding and Kanaan, 2016). Hospitals are relatively strange places, with communal wards, unfamiliar sights, sounds and smells, and strange nomenclature.

3.   The medical problem means that some forms of intervention become imperative (e.g. Ziebland et al., 2015). In acute-care settings the medical problem dominates and sometimes it necessitates urgent treatment. Whilst the patient expects to be consulted and retains the right to withhold consent to treatment, there is much less scope for the patient to negotiate treatment options.

In acute care, the priority nursing work is directed at the medical problem. The patient is stabilised, protected from imminent additional threats, and it is only later that care is deliberated upon more in personal choice terms. Abraham's case study (Chapter 3) is an example of this sort of situation. The patient is threatened by a severe Covid-19 infection illness. He requires emergency treatment that potentially will save his life but which has sequelae of its own. Abraham has to learn to mobilise again afterwards, and this happens whilst he is still making sense of the dilemma. Pre-planned surgery in the acute-care setting offers greater scope for patient consultation and partnership (see Chapter 4, John's case study), but even here a medical imperative exists for surgery. Without a resection of the tumour, it is likely that the bowel cancer will spread locally and metastasise, causing more significant risks for the patient. So, whilst the patient is afforded an excellent preparation and supported with skill, the medical imperative remains. Particular treatment is required, dictated by pathology and not by insights into the patient's personal world.

Within longer-term care relationships there is considerably more scope to address the problems through what is learned from a patient narrative. Greater choice becomes possible, for instance not only with regard to how care is experienced, but also which treatment options are used. It becomes possible to examine the medical problem through the lens of the personal problem, the way in which the patient perceives their circumstances and needs. Tom's case study (Chapter 5) and Susan's case study (Chapter 6) become clearly more consultative and negotiated in nature. The patient has much greater scope to negotiate care decisions and plans using what they know about themselves and about the treatment options available. In such settings there is often more self-care work for the patient to do, and with the responsibilities there come additional opportunities as regards the design of the care planned.

Activity 7.2   Speculating

Pause briefly now to speculate upon what person-centred care in the acute-care setting might centre upon.

Jot your ideas down before reading on to my reflections that follow.

I believe that person-centred care is still possible within the acute-care setting, however. The patient's concerns linked to acute and sometimes sudden illness may centre much less upon co-designing care and much more upon securing prompt and effective treatment. The patient usually trusts in the expertise of the clinician, nurse or doctor, and expects them to work within strict clinical guidelines and standards designed to protect the patient's best interests (Turnbull et al., 2018). Negotiated care, with shared decision-making responsibilities that attend that, is something that grows as urgent threats recede and equilibrium is secured.

Person-centred care might focus upon rather different things within the acute-care setting:

1. Helping the patient to manage the anxiety that typically attends hospital treatment (e.g. Webster et al., 2017). The nurse works to make the strange environment less threatening and more accessible as regards what the clinicians propose. The nurse explains the investigative process – that necessary to secure a clear diagnosis.

2. Protecting the patient, advocating his or her interests and concerns and ensuring that as far as is practicable consent to treatment or care measures is truly informed (Peterson et al., 2019). In acute care the nurse acts as the patient's advocate, helping to rebalance power where clinicians know more than the patient does.

3. Promoting patient dignity (Lin and Tsai, 2019). This is much more than simply ensuring that the patient is adequately attired, addressed with respect and handled gently. It extends into the patient's need to story their experiences to others, staff, friends or relatives. Patients need to be able to narrate what is being done in ways that preserve their sense of integrity. Patients need incrementally more information, and they need help to rehearse it in ways that make personal sense.

This is vitally important work if the patient is to manage the challenge of admission to hospital. Successful communication serves not only to inform the patient and secure consent, but also to help them narrate the experience as, on balance, beneficial.

In the acute-care setting the early-stage relationship work is of particular concern. Nurses need to anticipate the sorts of needs and concerns that patients will have when they come to hospital. But nurses also have to stand ready to augment the understanding of concerns when the patient is then met. Relating to the patient is very important; we need to establish rapport when the patient feels vulnerable. This means that we have to learn to secure and interpret patient narratives very quickly indeed. The patient narrative may be fragmented and jumbled, but every effort has to be made to understand what the patient is experiencing and what opening sense they make of this (Egerod et al., 2020). The ability to listen attentively is at least as important as the ability to explain what is happening to the patient. Negotiating care – collaborating and evaluating upon it – is important too, but there may be much less scope for you to exercise skills there, at least until the patient has taken stock and started to recover their equilibrium. Notice in Abraham's case study (Chapter 3) how the bulk of that work was done on the rehabilitation ward, after Abraham had spent time in intensive care.

In longer-term care relationships there is greater scope for the traditional interpretation of person-centred care to be expressed. There the nurse can build through the care relationship stages in the sequence envisaged. Care needs are anticipated and then the nurse meets the patient and begins a mutual investigative and planning process with them. There is ample time to build a rapport with the patient and often much greater rationale for the patient to adopt a collaborative role, partnering the nurse as hoped. Nothing persuades the patient to adopt an active care-partnering role more than the realisation that without self-care work, significant problems are likely to arise almost immediately.

Person-centred care skill development

This raises the question about what it takes to practise person-centred care in a successful way. You might have already met nurses who think and act in truly person-centred ways, but it might be harder to understand how they did that. We need to review what skills are required to practise this way and now, at the end of the book, to deliberate on which you would like to develop more in the future. Let's proceed through the different stages of the care relationship to detail the skill requirements.

Anticipating care requirements

I wonder if you were struck in this book by just how important research and other forms of evidence were in delivering person-centred care. Evidence is understood in its widest sense, the nurse reviewing and making sense of case study, audit and research-evidence insights. To practise person-centred care well, you need to be well prepared and to have amassed and reviewed a range of evidence about the patient's illness and their likely needs. You will need evidence not only about the 'hard facts' of disease or treatment options, but also about the human experience of different illnesses or injuries. If you work with children or elderly patients, you will need to understand how human development helps shape that information. Your nursing course is likely to teach you a great deal about accessing, reading and evaluating research evidence. Textbooks can teach you how to think more critically (e.g. Price, 2021). But you might quickly realise that the realm of evidence is vast; it is also a place of gaps and contradictions. Evidence can be fragmentary, inconsistent, so we have to acknowledge the limitations of knowledge.

I believe that nurses need to specialise to a significant degree when delivering person-centred care. It is unrealistic to command a wide range of evidence about many different patient groups and their needs and illnesses. It seems likely that the most successful person-centred care nurses work with very familiar, relatively circumscribed fields of practice. In an undergraduate nursing course that could seem daunting because you move through different placements. Later, though, you can commit to a chosen field of practice and read in depth about the clientele of patients that you serve there.

Relating to the person

Students tell me that this seems the most magical skill of expert nurses. Experts seem to know how to say the right things, in the right way and at the right time. This skill stems from understanding patient narratives. Each of the case studies in this book relied to a significant degree upon interpreting the narratives of patients. Without such access and understanding, it is impossible to deliver person-centred care. My conversations with clinicians have led me to believe that the rapport work done at the start of the care relationship comes down to four key things:

1. Conveying a sincere interest in the patient's experiences and concerns, typically through an invitation to recount what has been happening. We have to resist the rush to inform patients about what will be done. We have to accept that storytelling and listening is vital.

2. Encouraging the patient to recount events in their own terms. The nurse must accept the importance of perceptions, for it is on these that the patient often acts. A nurse establishes what a need is not only by what the patient describes as anxiety-provoking, but also through what the nurse knows may yet come in terms of investigations and treatment options. We name problems; we conceptualise them, for instance, as 'fears about insulin'. This skill is best achieved beside a skilled nurse who thinks aloud about what she or he has heard the patient say. If you see this as something that you would like to work upon much more, then a good way forward is to inform your practice supervisor you wish to work alongside nurses who seem especially adept at thinking aloud. Ask such skilled nurses to review with you case study care that you have been involved in. By talking about patient narratives, you will then develop greater confidence in building trust relationships with patients.

3. Checking that we have understood what the patient explained by feeding back brief summaries of what the patient has said. In many ways this is a familiar communication skill, but doing it fluently, authentically is important ('let's just summarise what seems of concern').

4. Summarising other narratives; what we have learned about need from past patients. Expert nurses do this rather a lot, of course protecting the identity of past confidantes, but still conveying insights into worries that convince the current patient that you understand a great deal about their own problems.

Activity 7.3   Reflection

Review now the above four skills that seem integral to relating to patients. How well developed are your skills here? Can you identify one or more experienced nurses that you would like to consult in future about such skills, perhaps discussing excerpts from your portfolio? Talking about talk is important and entirely valid nursing study work.

As this answer is based on your own reflection, no outline answer is given at the end of the chapter.

Negotiating person-centred care

In Chapter 2, I characterised negotiation as explaining risks, issues and problems, exploring possible goals of care, identifying options, clarifying expected contributions, and recording the plan of care. Looking back over the case studies, I realise that the skills associated with negotiating were developed in varying degrees. Talking to my correspondent case study nurses about this afterwards, we identified several factors that make negotiating care more difficult than it at first seems. The first of these concerned realising patient expectations. Each of the nurses admitted to a concern that patients might expect more of care than was realistically possible. The nurses explained that more assertive, insistent patients or relatives might secure more service than others and that this raised ethical questions. This remains a persistent concern in nursing and something that potentially undermines the partnership philosophy of care that we usually hope to promote. It is possible that a patient might demand a great deal and offer little contribution themself.

What seemed to support a more honest negotiation, though, was a clear set of principles about what a service could provide and a frank appraisal of the merits of patient contributions to care, the development of self-care facility. The health service, no matter how it is funded, is unequal to the plethora of demands that the public might expect. Of necessity, some needs have to be self-met. If you wonder about your negotiating skills, it is a good idea to first review what your local healthcare service commits to – the range of treatment and support options that are available. It is then wise to review what additional support options might be available, either through charitable organisations and support groups, or through supplementary purchased provision. As one of my correspondent case study nurses observed, 'you cannot be ashamed of what is possible if you are not resourced to address exceptional need. You have instead to confront managers with consistently expressed patient concerns and to explore ways in which patients and or relatives might be able to contribute more themselves'.

One of the problems of negotiating care is that nurses sometimes start with idealistic standards of care provision that significantly outstrip what the service commits to provide. Care *should* be like this. Nevertheless, the NMC code of conduct (NMC, 2018) makes it clear that we should recognise our skill and other limitations. We cannot commit to that which is beyond our skill level or available resources of the service. The individual nurse cannot pretend to always bridge the divide between sought care and equitable care in reality. One case study nurse correspondent said, 'you have to be frank with some patients. Fewer of them than you expect demand the earth. But if you fear that many might, then you fail to explore felt needs, to identify areas where you need to negotiate what *is* possible. So find out first what is feasible within service policies and guidelines, what you can recommend the patient source elsewhere if you cannot assist. You will then negotiate to better effect'.

Collaborating on person-centred care

I thought that all of the nurses in the case studies shared in this book adopted distinctive roles – that which were valuable in terms of patient support, but also seemed sustaining and motivating for the nurses themselves. The nurses were able to do this because they evaluated what they felt good at. 'I am pretty good at listening and counselling'; 'I like to explain or to teach'. It seems unlikely to me that at the end of your course in nursing you will have mastered every role and associated skill that is possible within person-centred care. Undergraduate education is much more about establishing the essential skills and securing insights into more advanced skills. Take heart, then – learning continues post-registration.

The obvious example here is the skill of teaching. If you master the skill of teaching, then your care reach extends much further into the realm of person-centred care. This is because you help create a learning opportunity for the patient. Just as you commit to teaching something, so the patient commits to learning something in turn. That might involve the patient in enquiring further about their illness, it might mean mastering a skill such as insulin therapy, but it creates a clear responsibility for sustaining an active patient role in the delivery of jointly made care plans.

Teaching begins with understanding what the patient needs to learn and then comparing that against their felt and expressed needs. Does the patient realise that they need to master something? Does the patient understand that their success in the face of illness or injury might depend upon successful learning? If expressed needs are wildly different to the need to learn something, then it becomes necessary to say to the patient that they may face a problem ahead.

When we reviewed the list of skills linked to collaborating on care, two of my correspondents highlighted the importance of monitoring patient and relationship progress. The first explained to me that written care plans were sometimes the briefest summaries of the care relationship and shared goals. The shared plans developed apace, dependent on what the patient discovered was either easy or difficult. Securing a patient commitment to a goal, what they would achieve as well as expect of the nurse, was sometimes difficult. This was because care was iterative and closely referenced experiences met along the way. Chloe (Chapter 5) explained that what followed on from an experiential day learning about diabetes self-care depended on what patient and parent then reported about their experiences. Monitoring was important then; rechecking experiences of 'work done together'. As Chloe explained, 'informed consent is an ongoing, felt thing. The patient does, or doesn't, feel able to carry on committing to the work. So you might write up periodic updates on the same, but day-to-day care collaboration work is much harder to record in the classic goal, activity, timescale form'.

Evaluating person-centred care

Of all the care relationship stages shared within the four case studies of this book, evaluating person-centred care was the most mercurial. Sometimes the evaluations were entirely uplifting, for instance as a patient described her recovery from depression (Susan, Chapter 6). At other times, however, it was difficult to judge how secure patient progress really was. Abraham (Chapter 3), for instance, clearly had discoveries still to make about his progress when he returned home to his wife. Confidence levels depended upon the challenges that emerged, and some of those were likely to arise later. So, two of the challenges of evaluating person-centred care concern deciding when to pause and to take stock, and then how to describe that appraisal. Is it an interim evaluation? Is a great deal more progress possible later on if we wait rather longer to judge progress? A patient might initially observe that they feel extremely content with that achieved, only to revise the judgement later if new challenges emerged. We have to judge when to determine what the outcome was.

Some ambiguity also remains as regards the focus of evaluation within person-centred care, at least concerning the four case studies here. In ideal form the evaluation is 360 degrees, the patient evaluating their own work as well as support provided by the nurse. Both might report achievements, problems and discoveries associated with the process of negotiating care and sharing responsibilities there. But patients can be accustomed to evaluating service provision. Much evaluation conducted by healthcare organisations operates in that way, asking about what we did for you rather than exploring what we achieved together. In some instances (for example, John, Chapter 4) it is rather more difficult to judge the success or otherwise of care. When a patient has a learning disability, it can be more difficult to articulate satisfaction with what was achieved. Some patients may simply express satisfaction in the hope that this is what the nurse hopes to hear. Helping them to articulate in greater detail what was good, indifferent or problematic in the care process can be difficult indeed. In these circumstances it is often necessary to evaluate care together with the patient's advocate, working with someone who knows more about how the service user habitually copes, and what signals a sense of security and equilibrium.

Activity 7.4   Critical thinking

Even within the case studies of this book, person-centred care has some limitations. None of the correspondent nurses involved judged outcomes as entirely perfect. But I think that the case studies represent significant achievements. What do you think the case studies demonstrate about nursing skill, that which might have faltered had the person-centred care philosophy not guided the work?

An outline answer is given at the end of this chapter.

Enhancing future person-centred care

It is time briefly to look forward and to consider the future of person-centred care. Here I speculate on two changes that might enhance person-centred care – both significant, both aspirational. What might better facilitate person-centred care in the future? From a practitioner perspective, person-centred care is clearly attractive. It enables us to attend sensitively to patient need and quite often to articulate our skill and expertise (McCormack and McCance, 2017). In a conducive environment, person-centred care becomes much more satisfying work, something that we see empowers a patient. But as you will gather from the above, I think that there remain constraints upon its future expression.

Reconfiguring public expectation of the patient role

The most profound and beneficial change that might enhance person-centred care would involve a reconfiguration of public expectations of the patient role. Whilst this is a profound change, it is arguably necessary as we review the tensions between public expectations of the NHS and what seems realisable. Nursing faces a difficulty in this area because conceptions of the service have tended to focus on what clinicians will do for clients whilst nursing focuses on what can be collaborated upon (Mold, 2015; Latimer et al., 2017). The consumer has too often been conceived of as a relatively passive figure. In welfare state conceptions of healthcare provision, public expectations of the health service have incrementally outstripped what has been provided (Welch, 2018). No matter how cherished an institution the British NHS is, it has become a hostage to fortune. Debates about the distinction between social and nursing care have arisen in part because of the difficulty meeting public expectations of care. In health insurance-based healthcare systems, theoretically there is greater scope for more bespoke care, but realistically too that quickly collides with the insurance premiums that need to be paid (Niles, 2018). Those unable to afford significant premiums are cast back upon what can seem substandard care, which poses its own dilemmas for the ethos of nursing.

Imagine, however, a new social contract facilitated between the public and healthcare services, that which requires more of patient and/or relative input into care. What I commend here is not a withdrawal of care services, leaving precariously resourced patients with less support, but a greater emphasis on norm expectations of patients learning ways to self-care, to manage their health circumstances better than before. A revised contract between the public and the NHS could transform the work of nurses and specifically build better opportunities for person-centred care. The change would need to clarify a range of chronic illness circumstances where learning to self-care was established as the clear expectation, this as part of public education. If this was then coupled with a public health service drive to encourage prevention of chronic illnesses in the first place, there might then be clearer focus for person-centred care. Presumptions of partnering and shared care responsibilities would become expected in a range of chronic illness situations. Whilst patient capacity to partner is affected by many things, for example the ability to learn to self-care, starting with the assumption that more patient roles are active rather than passive would significantly improve the chances that nurses could work more imaginatively with patients. Where nurses have to rescue less, there is a chance for healthier outcomes to be achieved and for the health service to work in a more strategic way. Many patients are already motivated by personal protection or health improvement to liaise well with nurses, but the expectation of collaboration is arguably not as widespread as it should be.

Activity 7.5   Investigation

Access now via the internet the article below on healthcare consumerism by Iliffe and Manthorpe (2020). This free-to-access article traces the history of healthcare consumer thinking and how that has been viewed in medicine. It has its most obvious application in healthcare systems where patients privately purchase healthcare and compare options available. Here, though, I encourage you to read it with regard to the possibilities for patient–clinician partnering. You see, informed consumership empowers patients with knowledge that they could contribute to care partnerships and an increased self-care responsibility. But consumership might too simply lead to more strident demands of healthcare services.

Reflect now with your colleagues which seems more likely. If you favour more partnership work, how might you, in your setting, argue for that as a better way forward?

Iliffe, S and Manthorpe, J (2020) Medical consumerism and the modern patient: successful ageing, self-management and the 'fantastic prosumer'. *Journal of the Royal Society of Medicine, 113* (9): 339–45. doi: 10.1177/0141076820911574

As this answer is based on your own reflection, no outline answer is given at the end of the chapter.

Developing the teaching potential of healthcare staff

You will sense in this book that I am enthusiastic about patient education, placing learning at the centre of many care negotiations. Nurses, because of their frequently sustained contact with patients and their intimate interest in the experience of illness, deficit or injury, are well placed to act as teachers of patients. Many advanced and specialist practitioner roles already have a significant educational role and many nurses enjoy teaching. Patient education has the potential to not only liberate patients from a range of problems but also to protect hard-pressed healthcare services against at least some recurring costs (for example, when patients are hospitalised for repeated chronic illness problems). A strategy needs to be developed with regard to which nurses teach, how much education figures in acute versus rehabilitation care and what essential skills are taught within the patient education part of the nursing syllabus (see Table 7.1 for possible examples).

Historically, much of the public teaching work of nursing was concentrated within public health settings and assigned to the work of health visitors. That work remains important but because it seems likely that despite public health endeavours, a variety of patients will still suffer chronic illnesses, there arises important patient education work to be completed. A significant amount of current nurse learning could contribute to patient education. That which we learn about as regards communication, reassurance, psychological support and rehabilitation, about explaining treatment and informed consent, could all play into a wider nurse education on the strategic use of teaching and the facilitation of learning. However, both of the speculated changes would need to work in train with the other. To partner effectively, both parties need to anticipate a role and quite often change requires learning.

Table 7.1 Possible components of patient education theme in the nursing syllabus

Teaching skill	Person-centred care relevance
Conceptualising learning work (what it takes to learn and adjust when ill)	Learning involves both cognitive (reasoning) and emotional effort and that varies dependent on the nature of illness and patient learning context. Some of the patient narrative will relate to the experience of learning.
Assessing learning styles and needs	People learn in individual ways, but we must still design education that is cost-efficient and effective as well. Nurses will need to assess what educational package best suits an individual patient.
Agreeing learning outcomes and then harnessing human motivation as part of learning	Patients vary as regards their confidence learning and they may focus on different things to sustain their study. As we monitor patient progress, we will need to understand why a patient excels or struggles whilst learning.
Designing learning resources and activities	The person-centred care nurse works creatively with patients to plan solutions to problems to meet needs. Person-centred care offers the chance to co-design learning activity with the patient.
Teaching activities (e.g. demonstrating, coaching)	Person-centred care nurses adopt different roles and use different activities to teach patients. Nurses need an appropriate techniques range.
Assessing learning achievements and insights	Patients are likely to be motivated by very individual needs and goals, so assessment measures will need to accommodate those.
Reviewing and improving educational designs	It would be inefficient if the person-centred care nurse constantly developed new teaching packages for every patient. The nurse will need to repurpose some of them.

If patient narratives are to become more optimistic and 'can do' in style, if they are to insulate the patient against future problems, then person-centred care nurses will need further assistance on how best to teach patients. Excellent education not only explains an illness or a treatment regimen, it also suggests ways to think about and solve problems, to increase personal control over health and lifestyle irrespective of the illness suffered. The purpose of the teacher is to liberate the reasoning of the learner, to increase their independence. This ethos operates in the same way that the person-centred care nurse works to liberate the patient from their dependence on nursing care and to a significant extent the rescue services of the NHS. The more that the patient has control of their own circumstances, the command of coping resources, the less they are likely to need a nurse or a doctor to respond on their behalf.

Chapter summary

We have now reached the end of this chapter and indeed the book as a whole. I want to thank the nurses who kindly shared their case studies with me and the debates and discussions about person-centred care that emerged through each. What I hope you will take away from this chapter and the discussions before is an increasing enthusiasm for and confidence in your ability to explain and to demonstrate person-centred care work.

To practise in a person-centred way, we need to find ways to explain the approach to ourselves and others. Importantly, that explanation needs to be realisable in nursing care today. As this book has demonstrated, person-centred care cannot operate abstractly as a philosophy; it has to work with the system in which nurses practise. Person-centred care is not the only approach to nursing, but it has a vital part to play. The NMC code of conduct (NMC, 2018) makes clear and repeated reference to the need to personalise nursing care, working with the patient to ensure that we address their needs and circumstances. Making person-centred care real, however, making it operational, means that we have to better articulate the stages of the care relationship and the skills that are required to deliver care in a person-centred way. This chapter has highlighted just what improvements within the healthcare system might facilitate that, which might enable nurses to demonstrate person-centred care in its fullest sense.

Where you practise may set limits on person-centred care, but as the case studies in this book have illustrated, there is always scope to help the patient to feel dignified. Much of what person-centred care becomes in the future depends not just upon nursing philosophy but also upon the review and improvement of healthcare services. Much of what we do will necessarily work with how patients conceive of their roles, and critically, how they hope to liaise with nurses to address their healthcare needs. Nurses should stand ready to help influence the direction of change, for much of what seems sustainable and meaningful in our work depends upon how patients and systems conceive of nursing's contribution.

Activities: Brief outline answers

Activity 7.1 Reflection (p157)

One of the key determinants of whether person-centred care thrives in a particular environment is the prevailing attitude towards communication. If enquiry is conceived of largely in terms of an opening patient history (open enquiry) but then predominantly closed-question checks on understanding of/satisfaction with recommended care (those eliciting yes or no answers), there is much less scope for person-centred care.

Person-centred care requires regular open-enquiry conversations so that the patient's narrative is re-accessed and understood afresh. Historically, a manager might have cautioned junior colleagues to not 'gossip' with the patients. But therapeutic conversation is quite different, focusing on patient experience and perceived need. You can check then on the person-centred care potential of a setting by the extent to which care includes therapeutic communication. The pressure of medical interventions, shorter hospital stays for patients and often heavy physical workloads all combine to limit person-centred care in acute-care settings, but they should not block our commitment to hearing what the patient says and attending to their concerns.

Activity 7.4 Critical thinking (p164)

I was greatly encouraged by the nurses' skills exhibited in the case studies, even if my correspondents felt that care could have been even better. In Abraham's case study the nurses show considerable skill anticipating Abraham's most urgent needs and summarising what treatment and care will assist him with the same. The fact that such needs are recurring and common to many patients suffering from severe Covid-19 infection is, I think, immaterial. Abraham's anxiety was understood and addressed. Later, the rehabilitation work was justified with regard to his need to return home to care for his wife. There was a clear appreciation of risk and an understanding too of how to build the patient's confidence levels.

I think what impresses about John's case study was the liaison work done to ensure that John's hospital stay was as stress-free as possible. Both healthcare professionals are making strategic use of evidence and other information to design care for the patient and then checking that the proposed ideas feel workable for the patient. The investment within this passage of care was considerable, but it was arguably well chosen given that the patient would require two operations and possibly (in the future) other treatment for bowel cancer. So, care was strategic and well justified.

In Tom's case study I identified skills of diplomacy, insights into teenage-years psychology and a good understanding of motivation. The nurse is already an accomplished teacher who through her role has the opportunity to facilitate learning in different ways. This more eclectic teaching plan looks time-expensive in terms of the nurse as a service resource, but it seems well justified given that the needs of two patients were addressed through the planned day.

In Susan's case study the nurse showed considerable organisational skills and those associated with interprofessional practice. The patient's developing narrative was understood and work was undertaken to conceive of a rehabilitation plan that met the patient's needs and which helped a GP become more confident combining therapies. The benefits from this case study may well advantage other patients that follow afterwards.

Further reading

Ku, B and Lupton, E (2020) *Health Design Thinking: Creating Products and Services for Better Health.* New York: Cooper Hewitt.

When you begin to doubt that we can help patients secure more control of their lives and convince them that they can manage chronic illness well, this is a go-to reassurance book. The case study innovations are often technological and tool-based, but the 'can-do' thinking is refreshing.

Sassen, B (2018) *Nursing: Health Education and Improving Patient Self-Management.* Cham, Switzerland: Springer International.

This book conflates what we think of as health promotion with illness self-care learning, but no matter, it is a valuable follow-up read if you are interested in teaching as a means of helping patients to improve their lot.

Stirk, S and Sanderson, H (2012) *Person-Centred Organisations: Strategies and Tools for Managing Change in Health, Social Care and the Voluntary Sector.* London: Jessica Kingsley.

There is a paucity of good books on how to arrange healthcare services in more person-centred ways, so I have no qualms about recommending this older text to you. The challenges remain surprisingly constant: that associated with bespoke versus generic care and that associated with resource management and enthusing healthcare staff.

Glossary of key terms

anticipating care   The preparatory work that a nurse does by reading research, audit, case study and other materials to better understand the possible needs of patients that come into their care.

attribution theory   The notion that we habitually assign meanings to experiences and endeavours, creating a sense of purpose and sometimes pleasure en route. Attribution theory is important as a means of explaining motivation.

collaborating   The delivery of person-centred care; the sharing of experiences and activities that are jointly seen as beneficial and which work towards agreed goals.

discourse   A positional statement or series of arguments that express our values or our understanding of events. So, within nursing, there is a discourse about what person-centred care should look like. In palliative care there is a discourse associated with end-of-life care. Discourses compete and clash within healthcare, making it harder for us to know how best to proceed. To support a discourse, we need to understand the underpinning premises and the values and beliefs that are attached.

empowering/empowerment   Enabling patients to take increasing control and responsibility regarding their illness and associated needs. It is furthered by sharing information, building confidence and enabling the patient to learn.

evaluating   The process of summarising what has been learned and achieved through collaborative activity. Evaluation may be interim (judging progress) or summative (judging the care at completion).

medical problem   The challenge posed by injury or disease and which might create several imperative demands for treatment (see also personal problem).

motivation   That which sustains individuals in their efforts and that which makes activities meaningful. Understanding motivation is important if patients are to learn well and to maintain self-care in adverse circumstances. There are different ways of describing motivation. It may be driven by a search for rewards, or by an increasing sense of purpose linked to meaningful activities that help confirm a satisfying identity.

narrative   A story or explanation embedded within a series of words; the dialogues shared with others. The narrative may convey how we see ourselves, how we cope with illness, or (as a nurse or lay carer) how we try to care. Narratives may be hidden. Sometimes the nurse has to check carefully what patients are in fact conveying in their narrative.

negotiating   The process of jointly deliberating on the possibilities of the care relationship; what needs to be done, who might take responsibility for work and which roles might be adopted.

PERSON   A mnemonic to help nurses remember what shapes person-centred nursing care. A focus on Perception and a willingness to Explore experiences through narratives; the need to Relate to the patient's perceptions and to Source the origins of their worries, what might sustain hope; the nurse Outlines a plan with the patient and then will Notify all those asked to assist.

personal problem   The experience of illness or injury as couched within a person's individual context. The medical problem is understood and narrated through a personal circumstance and experience (see also medical problem).

person-centred care (pragmatic)   Care that centres on the person within a healthcare system that sets significant limits on resources, and which serves the many as well as the individual. Pragmatic person-centred care elucidates role responsibilities for the nurse and the patient, acknowledging the expertise that the nurse brings to bear in the service of the patient (see also Chapter 1).

personhood   That which distinguishes us as whole and different from others. The person is defined by their abilities and aptitudes, by their attitudes and values, and through the relationships they share with others. Illness and treatment may undermine personhood through its impact on the body and on our sense of control over daily living.

rapport   A mutual state of respect and understanding, where each understands and appreciates the contribution of the other.

relating   The second stage of person-centred care where the nurse and the patient meet and explore expectations of one another and the care that might be shared.

role   In person-centred care, both nurses and patients adopt roles, the better to effect a plan of care. For example, the nurse might play the role of teacher and the patient learner, or, indeed, when the patient is the expert of managing a chronic illness, vice versa.

standard care   A largely pre-set package of care based upon assessment of the medical problem and commonly arising needs. Standard care packages recognise the challenges of delivering equitable care to all, a transparent commitment to minimum provision.

templates   Human beings develop working templates (summary explanations) to explain experience and endeavour. Exploring a narrative often reveals such templates so that the nurse and patient can review whether the same are beneficial.

therapeutic relationship   That which describes how the nurse and patient relate to one another in ways that achieve beneficial ends. To be therapeutic, the nurse musters communication and clinical skills and makes selective use of evidence to guide the patient. The relationship extends to become a culture where a wide range of staff and services are marshalled so as to advance the needs of the individual patient.

References

Albert, J (2015) *Problem Solving Strategies: Decision Making.* Scotts Valley, CA: Create Space Independent Publishing.

Alshmemri, M, Shahwan-Akl, L and Maude, P (2017) Herzberg's two-factor theory. *Life Science Journal, 14* (5): 12–16.

Anderson, C and Tapesh, R (2013) Patient experiences of taking antidepressants for depression: a secondary qualitative analysis. *Research in Social and Administrative Pharmacy, 9* (6): 884–902.

Anuradha, S (2015) Effect of a structured teaching programme on prevention of hypoglycaemia among diabetic patients. *International Journal of Nursing Education, 7* (4): 47–52.

Avery, A, Whitehead, K and Halliday, V (2016) *How to Facilitate Lifestyle Change: Applying Group Education in Healthcare.* Chichester: Wiley Blackwell.

Backman, A, Ahnlund, P, Sjogren, K et al. (2019) Embodying person-centred being and doing: leading towards person-centred care in nursing homes as narrated by managers. *Journal of Clinical Nursing, 29* (1–2). doi: 10.1111/jocn.15075

Bastable, S (2017) *Nurses as Educators: Principles of Teaching and Learning for Nursing Practice* (5th edition). London: Jones and Bartlett.

Blair, J, Anthony, T, Gunther, I et al. (2017) A protocol for the preparation of patients for theatre and recovery. *Learning Disability Practice, 20* (2): 22–6.

Brittan, N, Moore, L, Lydhal, D et al. (2016) Elaboration of the Gothenburg model of person-centred care. *Health Expectations, 20*: 407–18.

Brokerhof, I, Yberna, J and Bal, M (2020) Illness narratives and chronic patients' sustainable employability: the impact of positive work stories. *PLoS One, 15* (2). doi: 10.1371/journal.pone.0228581

Brown, M, Chouliara, Z, MacArthur, J et al. (2016) The perspectives of stakeholders of intellectual disability liaison nurses: a model of compassionate, person-centred care. *Journal of Clinical Nursing, 25* (7–8): 972–82.

Brown, R, Barbour, P and Martin, D (2015) *The Mental Capacity Act 2005: A Guide for Practice* (3rd edition). London: SAGE/Learning Matters.

Brown, T and Ladwig, S (2020) Covid-19, China and the World Health Organization, and the limits of international health diplomacy. *American Journal of Public Health, 110* (8): 1149–51.

Buckley, C, McCormack, B and Ryan, A (2018) Working in a storied way: narrative-based approaches to person-centred care and practice development in older adult residential care settings. *Journal of Clinical Nursing, 27* (5–6). doi: 10.1111/jocn.14201

Byrne, A, Baldwin, A and Harvey, C (2020) Whose centre is it anyway? Defining person-centred care in nursing: an integrative review. *PLoS One, 15* (3): e0229923.

Carter, L, Read, J, Pyle, M et al. (2018) 'I believe I know better even than the psychiatrists what caused it': exploring the development of causal beliefs in people experiencing psychosis. *Community Mental Health Journal, 54* (6): 805–13.

Chinn, D and Homeyard, C (2017) Easy-read and accessible information for people with intellectual disabilities: is it worth it? A meta narrative literature review. *Health Expectations, 20* (6): 1189–1200.

Christie, J, Mitchell, W and Marshall, M (2020) *Promoting Resilience in Dementia Care: A Person-Centred Framework for Assessment and Support Planning.* London: Jessica Kingsley.

Conklin, L and Strunk, D (2015) A session-to-session examination of homework engagement in cognitive therapy for depression: do patients experience immediate benefits? *Behavioural Research and Therapy, 72*: 56–62.

Corbett, A (2019) *Intellectual Disability and Psychotherapy: The Theories, Practice and Influence of Valerie Sinason.* Abingdon: Routledge.

Counselling Directory (2018) *Mental Health Facts and Figures.* Available online at: www.counselling-directory-org.uk/stats.html

Dagnan, D, Jackson, I and Eastlake, L (2018) A systematic review of cognitive behavioural therapy for anxiety in adults with intellectual disabilities. *Journal of International Disability Research, 62* (1): 974–91.

Dennis, C, Baxter, P, Ploeg, J et al. (2017) Models of partnership within family-centred care in the acute paediatric setting: a discussion paper. *Journal of Advanced Nursing, 73*(2). doi: 10.1111/jan.13178

Desmond Project (2018) *Developing Quality Structured Education in Diabetes.* Available online at: www.desmond.project.org.uk

Ding, J and Kanaan, R (2016) What should we say to patients with unexplained neurological symptoms? How explanation affects offence. *Journal of Psychosomatic Research, 91*: 55–60.

Doherty, M and Thompson, H (2014) Enhancing person-centred care through the development of the therapeutic relationship. *British Journal of Community Nursing, 19* (10): 504–7.

Donnelly, G (2012) Healthcare and the renaissance of holism. *Holistic Nursing Practice, 26* (3). doi: 10.1097/HNP.0b13e31824fe309

Dozeman, E, Van Marwijk, H, Van Schaik, D et al. (2012) Contradictory effects for prevention of depression and anxiety in residents in homes for the elderly: a pragmatic randomized controlled trial. *International Psychogeriatrics, 24* (8): 1242–51.

Drozd, M and Clinch, C (2016) The experiences of orthopaedic and trauma nurses who have cared for adults with a learning disability. *International Journal of Orthopaedic and Trauma Nursing, 22*: 13–23.

Egerod, I, Bogeskov, B, Jensen, J et al. (2020) Narrative critical care: a literary analysis of first-person critical illness pathographies. *Journal of Critical Care, 59*: 194–200.

Ellis, P (2019) *Evidence-Based Practice in Nursing* (4th edition). London: SAGE.

Elwyn, G, Edwards, A and Thompson, A (2016) *Shared Decision Making in Healthcare: Achieving Evidence-Based Patient Choice.* Oxford: Oxford University Press.

Etkind, S, Bristowe, K, Bailey, K et al. (2016) How does uncertainty shape patient experience in advanced illness? A secondary analysis of qualitative data. *Palliative Medicine, 31* (2). doi: 10.1177/0269216316647610.

Fathi, N and Rezaei, N (2020) Lymphopenia in COVID-19: therapeutic opportunities. *Cell Biology International, 44* (9): 1792–7.

Feldman, R, Dunner, D, Muller, J et al. (2013) Medicare patient experience with vagus nerve stimulation for treatment resistant depression. *Journal of Medical Economics, 16* (1): 62–74.

Frank, L, Matza, L, Handon, J et al. (2007) The patient experience of depression and remission: focus group results. *Journal of Nervous and Mental Disease, 195* (8): 647–54.

Galanti, G (2015) *Caring for Patients from Different Cultures* (5th edition). Philadelphia, PA: University of Pennsylvania Press.

Galliher, R, McLean, K and Syed, M (2017) An integrated developmental model for studying identity content in context. *Developmental Psychology, 53* (11): 2011–19.

Gandhi, R, Lynch, J and de Rio, C (2020) Mild and moderate Covid-19. *New England Journal of Medicine.* doi: 10.1056/NEJMep2009249

Garrouste-Orgeas, M, Flahault, C, Vinatier, I et al. (2019) Effect of an ICU diary on posttraumatic stress disorder symptoms among patients receiving mechanical ventilation: a randomized clinical trial. *JAMA: Journal of the American Medical Association, 322* (3): 229–239.

Ginicola, M, Smith, C and Trzaska, J (2015) Counseling through images: using photography to guide the counseling process and achieve treatment goods. *Journal of Creativity in Mental Health, 7* (4): 310–29.

Goldman, S, Brettle, A and McAndrew, S (2016) A client focused perspective of the effectiveness of Counselling for Depression (CfD). *Counselling and Psychotherapy Research, 16* (4): 288–97.

Gomez-Urquiza, J, Hueso-Montoro, G, Urquiza-Olmo, J et al. (2016) A randomized controlled trial of the effect of a photographic display with and without music on pre-operative anxiety. *Journal of Advanced Nursing, 72* (7): 1666–76.

Graner, K, Rolim, G, Moraes, A et al. (2016) Feelings, perceptions and expectations of patients during the process of oral cancer diagnosis. *Supportive Care in Cancer, 24* (5). doi: 10.1007/s00520-015-3030-0

Griemas, A (1983) *Structural Semantics.* Lincoln, NE: University of Nebraska Press.

Griscti, O, Aston, M, Martin-Misener, R et al. (2016) The experiences of chronically ill patients and registered nurses when they negotiate patient care in hospital settings: A feminist poststructural approach. *Journal of Clinical Nursing.* doi: 10.1111/jocn.13250

Grohmann, B, Espin, S and Gucciardi, E (2017) Patients' experiences of diabetes education teams' integration into primary care. *Canadian Family Physician, 63* (2): e128–e136.

Gulanick, M and Myers, J (2017) *Nursing Care Plans: Diagnoses, Interventions and Outcomes* (9th edition). Edinburgh: Elsevier.

Haake, R (2017) Counselling for depression: efficient, effective and evidence-based. *Healthcare Counselling and Psychotherapy Journal, 17* (4). Available online at: www.bacp. co.uk/bacp-journals/healthcare-counselling-and-psychotherapy-journal/october-2017/counselling-for-depression

Hansen, T, Zwisler, A, Berg, S et al. (2016) Cardiac rehabilitation patients' perspectives on their recovery following heart valve surgery: a narrative analysis. *Journal of Advanced Nursing.* doi: 10.1111/jan.12904

Harrison, J, Garrido, A, Rhymas, S et al. (2017) New institutionalization following acute hospital admission: a retrospective cohort study. *Age and Ageing, 46* (2): 238–44.

Hashem, M, Nelliot, A and Needham, D (2016) Early mobilization and rehabilitation in the ICU: moving back to the future. *Respiratory Care, 61* (7): 971–9.

Havaei, F, MacPhee, M and Dahinton, S (2019) The effect of nursing care delivery models on quality and safety outcomes of care: a cross sectional survey of medical-surgical nurses. *Journal of Advanced Nursing.* doi: 10.111/jan.13997

Heaslip, V and Bruce, L (2019) *Research and Evidence-Based Practice: For Nursing, Health and Social Care Students.* London: Lantern Press.

Heffer, T and Willoughby, T (2017) A count of coping strategies: a longitudinal study investigating an alternative method to understanding coping and adjustment. *PLoS One.* doi: 10.1371/journal.pone.0186057

Hermans, H, Wieland, J, Jelluma, N et al. (2013) Reliability and validity of the Dutch version of the Glasgow Anxiety Scale for people with an intellectual disability (GAS-ID). *Journal of Intellectual Disability Research, 57* (8): 728–36.

Herzberg, F (1966) *Work and the Nature of Man.* New York: World Publishing.

Hoedemakers, M, Leijten, M, Looman, W et al. (2019) Integrated care of frail elderly: a qualitative study of a promising approach in the Netherlands. *International Journal of Integrated Care, 19* (3). doi: 10.5334/ijic.4626

Hollins, S, Avis, A, Cheverton, S et al. (2015) *Going to Hospital.* London: Books Beyond Words.

Hopton, A, Eldred, J and MacPherson, H (2014) Patients' experiences of acupuncture and counselling for depression and comorbid pain: a qualitative study nested within a randomized controlled trial. *BMJ Open, 4:* e005144: doi: 10.1136/bmjopen-2014-00514-4

Horigan, G, Davies, M, Findlay-White, F et al. (2017) Systematic review or meta-analysis: reasons why patients referred to diabetes education programmes choose not to attend – systematic review. *Diabetic Medicine, 34* (1): 14–26.

Iliffe, S and Manthorpe, J (2020) Medical consumerism and the modern patient: successful ageing, self-management and the 'fantastic prosumer'. *Journal of the Royal Society of Medicine, 113* (9): 339–45.

Jakhmola, S, Indari, O, Kashyap, D et al. (2020) Recent updates on Covid-19: a holistic review. *Heliyon.* doi: 10.1016/j.heliyon.2020.e05706

Johnson, R (2020) Dexamethasone and the management of Covid-19. *British Medical Journal, 370.* doi: 10.1136/bjm.m2648

Jolley, J (2020) *Introducing Research and Evidence-Based Practice for Nursing and Healthcare Professionals* (3rd edition). London: Routledge.

Jones, S, McGarrah, M and Kahn, J (2019) Social and emotional learning: a principled science of human development in context. *Educational Psychologist, 54* (3): 129–144.

Kazantzis, N, Dattillo, F, Dobson, F et al. (2017) *The Therapeutic Relationship in Cognitive-Behavioral Therapy: A Clinician's Guide.* London: Guilford Publications.

Keefer, A, Kreiser, N, Singh, V et al. (2016) Intolerance of uncertainty predicts anxiety outcomes following CBT in youth with Autistic Spectrum Disorder. *Journal of Autism and Development Disorders, 47* (12): 3949–58.

Keller, K, Reangsing, C and Schneider, J (2020) Clinical presentation and outcomes of hospitalized adults with Covid-19: a systematic review. *Journal of Advanced Nursing.* doi: 10.1111/jan14558

Kelly, M, Morse, J, Stover, A et al. (2011) Describing depression: congruence between patient experiences and clinical assessments. *British Journal of Clinical Psychology, 50* (1): 46–66.

Kiernan, J, Mitchell, D, Stansfield, J et al. (2019) Mothers' perspectives on the lived experience of children with intellectual disability and challenging behaviour. *Journal of Intellectual Disabilities, 23* (2): 175–90.

King, J, O'Neil, B, Ramsey, P et al. (2019) Identifying patients' support needs following critical illness: a scoping review of the qualitative literature. *Critical Care, 23* (1). doi: 10.1186/s13054-019-2441-6

Kragh, M, Moller, D, Wihlborg, C et al. (2017) Experiences of wake and light therapy in patients with depression: a qualitative study. *International Journal of Mental Health Nursing, 26* (2): 170–80.

Latimer, T, Roscamp, J and Papanikitis, A (2017) Patient centredness and consumerism in healthcare: an ideological mess. *Journal of the Royal Society of Medicine, 110* (11): 425–7.

Launer, J (2018) *Narrative-Based Practice in Health and Social Care: Conversations Inviting Change* (2nd edition). Oxford: Routledge.

Laursen, D, Frølich, A and Christensen, U (2017a) Patients' perception of disease and experience with Type 2 diabetes patient education in Denmark. *Scandinavian Journal of Caring Sciences, 31* (4): 1039–47.

Laursen, D, Christensen, K, Christensen, U and Frølich, A (2017b) Assessment of short and long-term outcomes of diabetes patient education using the health education impact questionnaire (HeiQ). *BMC Research Notes, 10* (1): 213. doi: 10.1186/s13104-017-2536-6

Leaver, A, Wade, B, Vasavada, M et al. (2018) Fronto-temporal connectivity predicts ECT outcome in major depression. *Frontiers of Psychiatry, 9.* doi: 10.3389/fpsyt.2018.00092

Levy, A, Huang, C, Huang, A et al. (2018) Recent approaches to improve medication adherence in patients with coronary heart disease: progress towards a learning healthcare system. *Current Atherosclerosis Reports, 20* (1). doi: 10.1007/S/1883-018-0707-0

Lin, Y and Tsai, Y (2019) Development and validation of a dignity in care scale for nurses. *Nursing Ethics, 26* (7–8): 2467–81.

Linden-Carmichael, A, Dziak, J and Lanza, S (2019) Dynamic features of problematic drinking: alcohol use disorder/latent classes across ages 18–64. *Alcohol and Alcoholism, 54* (1): 97–103.

Lindgreen, P, Rolving, N, Nielsen, C et al. (2016) Interdisciplinary cognitive behavioral therapy as a part of lumbar spinal fusion surgery rehabilitation: experience of patients with chronic low back pain. *Orthopaedic Nursing, 35* (4): 238–47.

Maedo, A, Nabeya, D, Nagano, H et al. (2021) Prone position ventilation and femoro-femoral veno-venous extracorporeal membrane oxygenation for Covid-19 treatment. *Respiratory Case Reports, 9* (1): doi: 10.1002/rcr2.700

Mahdevi, A (2020) A brief review of interplay between vitamin D and angiotensin-converting enzyme 2: implications for a potential treatment for Covid-19. *Reviews in Medical Virology.* doi: 10.1002/rmv.2119

Maloney, S, Kolanowski, A, Van Haitsma, K et al. (2018) Person-centred assessment and care planning. *The Gerontologist, 58* (supplement 1): S32–S47.

Marx, E and Padmanabhan, P (2021) *Digital Transformation: How Consumerism, Technology and Pandemic Are Accelerating the Future.* Abingdon: Taylor and Francis (CRC Press imprint).

Maslow, A (1954) *Motivation and Personality.* New York. Harper Row.

McCormack, B (2021) *Negotiating Partnerships with Older People: A Person-Centred Approach.* London: Routledge.

McCormack, B and McCance, T (2017) *Person-Centred Practice in Nursing and Health Care: Theory and Practice* (2nd edition). Chichester: Wiley/Blackwell.

McKenna, H, Pajnkihar, M and Murphy, F (2014) *Fundamentals of Nursing Models, Theories and Practice* (2nd edition). Chichester: Blackwell.

Meleis, A (2018) *Theoretical Nursing: Development and Progress* (6th edition). New York: Wolters Kluwer Heath.

Mercer, C (2018) Primary care providers exploring value of 'social prescriptions' for patients. *Canadian Medical Association Journal, 190* (49): E1463–4.

Miller, M and Stoeckel, P (2017) *Client Education: Theory and Practice.* London: Jones and Bartlett Learning.

Mind (2018) *How Common Are Mental Health Problems?* Available online at: www.mind.org.uk/.../statistics.../how-common-are-mental-health-problems

Mintzberg, H (2017) *Managing the Myths of Healthcare: Bridging the Separations between Care, Cure, Control and Community.* Oakland, CA: Berrett-Kochler.

Mold, A (2015) *Making the Patient-Consumer: Patient Organisations and Health Consumerism in Britain.* Manchester: Manchester University Press.

Murphy, D (2019) *Person-Centred Experiential Counselling for Depression* (2nd edition). London: SAGE/BCAP.

Naldemirci, O, Britten, N, Lloyd, H and Wolf, A (2020) The potential and pitfalls of narrative elicitation in person-centred care. *Health Expectations, 23* (1): 238–46.

National Institute for Health and Care Excellence (NICE) (2009) *Depression in Adults: Recognition and Management.* Clinical Guideline (CG 90) updated April 2018. Available online at: www.nice.org.uk/search?q=cg90

Newton, M, Llewellyn, A and Hayes, S (2019) *The Care Process: Assessment, Planning, Implementation and Evaluation in Healthcare.* Banbury: Lantern Press.

Niles, N (2018) *Basics of the U.S. Health Care System.* London: Jones and Bartlett.

Noble, A, Mathieson, A, Ridsdale, L et al. (2019) Developing patient-centred, feasible alternative care for adult emergency department users with epilepsy: protocol for the mixed-methods observational 'collaborative' projects. *BMJ Open, 9* (11). doi: 10.1136/bmjopen-2019-031696

Northway, R, Rees, S, Davies, M and Williams, S (2017) Hospital passports, patient safety and person-centred care: a review of documents currently used for people with intellectual disabilities in the UK. *Journal of Clinical Nursing, 26* (23–4): 5160–8.

Nunstedt, H, Rudolfsson, G, Arlsen, P et al. (2017) Patients' variations of reflection about and understanding of long-term illness-impact of illness perception on trust in oneself and others. *The Open Nursing Journal, 11* (1): 43–53.

Nursing and Midwifery Council (NMC) (2018) *The Code: Professional Standards of Practice and Behaviour for Nurses, Midwives and Nursing Associates.* Available online at: www.nmc.org.uk/standards/code

Ocloo, J and Matthews, R (2015) From tokenism to empowerment: progressing patient and public involvement in healthcare improvement. *BMJ Quality and Safety, 25* (8). doi: 10.1136/bmjqs-2015-004839

Orem, D, Renpenning, K and Taylor, S (2003) *Self-Care Theory in Nursing: Selected Papers of Dorothea Orem.* Boston, MA: Springer.

Page, A and Stritzke, W (2015) Relating with clients, pp11–23 in *Clinical Psychology for Trainees: Foundations of Science Informed Practice* (2nd edition). Cambridge: Cambridge University Press.

Painter, J, Ingham, B, Trevithick, L et al. (2018) Correlates for the risk of specialist ID hospital admission for people with intellectual disabilities: development of the LDNAT inpatient index. *Tizard Learning Disability Review, 23* (1): 42–50.

Pasala, S, Barr, T and Messaoudi, I (2015) Impact of alcohol abuse on the adaptive immune system. *Alcohol Research, 37* (2): 185–97.

Pascarella, G, Strumia, A, Piliego, C et al. (2020) Covid-19 diagnosis and management: a comprehensive review. *Journal of Internal Medicine.* doi: 10.1111/joim.13091

Pate, J, Noblet, T, Hush, J et al. (2019) Exploring the concept of pain of Australian children with and without pain: a qualitative study. *BMJ Open, 9* (10). doi: 10.1136/bmjopen-2019-033199

Pauling, J, Reilly, E, Smith, T et al. (2018) 195 copers and catastrophists: coping strategies are associated with patient reported assessment of the severity and impact of Raynaud's phenomenon in systematic sclerosis. *Rheumatology, 57* (suppl. 3). doi: 10.1093/rheumatology/key075.419

Pearce, Z (2014) *Type 1 Diabetes: Causes, Treatment and Potential Complications.* New York: Nova Science Publishers.

Peterson, A, Berggarden, M, Schaller, A et al. (2019) Nurses' advocacy of clinical pain management in hospitals: a qualitative survey. *Pain Management Nursing, 20* (2): 133–9.

Pols, A, Schipper, K, Overkamp, D et al. (2017) Process evaluation of a stepped-care program to prevent depression in primary care: patients' and practice nurses' experiences. *BMC Family Practice, 18* (1): 26. doi: 10.1186/s12875-017-0583-7

Price, B (2015) Helping patients to learn about self-management. *Nursing Standard, 30* (2): 51–60.

Price, B (2016) Hallucinations: insights and supportive first care. *Nursing Standard, 30* (21): 49–60.

Price, B (2017) Developing patient rapport, trust and therapeutic relationships. *Nursing Standard, 31* (50): 52–63.

Price, B (2020) Ethical challenges in delivering person-centred care. *Primary Health Care, 30* (2): 34–41.

Price, B (2021) *Critical Thinking and Writing in Nursing* (5th edition). London: Learning Matters/SAGE.

Public Health England (2020) *Vaccine Update: Issue 315, December 2020, Covid-19 Special Edition.* London: UK Government.

Ratcliffe, M (2017) *Real Hallucinations: Psychiatric Illness, Intentionality and the Interpersonal World.* Boston, MA: MIT Press.

Renolen, A, Haye, S, Hjalmhult, E et al. (2018) 'Keeping on track': hospital nurses' struggles with maintaining workflow whilst seeking to integrate evidence-based practice into their daily work – a grounded theory study. *International Journal of Nursing Studies, 77*: 179–88.

Richards, B (2017) Caring for children with autism spectrum condition in paediatric emergency departments. *Emergency Nurse, 25* (4): 30–4.

Riding, S, Glendening, N and Heaslip, V (2017) Real world challenges in delivering person-centred care: a community-based case study. *British Journal of Community Nursing, 22* (8): 391–6.

Rogers, J and Maini, A (2016) *Coaching for Health: Why It Works and How to Do It.* Maidenhead: Open University Press.

Ross, T (2020) *Practical Budgeting for Health Care.* London: Jones and Bartlett.

Royal College of Psychiatrists (2009) *Antidepressants: Key Facts from the Royal College of Psychiatrists.* Available online at: www.rcpsych.ac.uk/pdf/antidepressants.pdf

Russell, B, Lincoln, C and Starkweather, A (2019) Distress tolerance intervention for improving self-management of chronic conditions: a systematic review. *Journal of Holistic Nursing, 37* (1): 74–86.

Saletnik, L (2019) Patients remember the little things. *AORN Journal, 109* (2): 153–4.

Salmon, N (2017) British people rank among the most depressed people in Western world. *The Independent,* 13 September. Available online at: www.independent.co.uk/news/uk/home-news/british-people-depression-west-mental-health-uk-oecd-europe-scandinavia-women-more-men-a7945321.html

Sanders, P and Hill, A (2014) *Counselling for Depression: A Person-Centred and Experiential Approach to Practice.* London: SAGE.

Sassen, B (2017) *Nursing: Health Education and Improving Self-Management.* New York: Springer.

Scheffelaar, A, Hendriks, M, Bos, N et al. (2019) Determinants of the quality of care relationships in long-term care: a participatory study. *BMC Health Services Research, 19* (1): 1–14.

Scheiner, G (2020) *Think Like a Pancreas: A Practical Guide to Managing Diabetes with Insulin* (3rd edition). New York: Hachette Go.

Schellinger, S, Anderson, E, Frazer, M et al. (2018) Patient self-defined goals: essentials of person-centred care for serious illness. *American Journal of Hospice and Palliative Medicine, 35* (1): 159–65.

Seavone, C, Brusco, S, Bertini, M et al. (2020) Current pharmacological treatments for Covid-19: what next? *British Journal of Pharmacology.* doi: 10.1111/bph.15072

Sekhon, M, Cartwright, M and Francis, J (2017) Acceptability of healthcare interventions: an overview of reviews and development of a theoretical framework. *BMC Health Services Research, 17* (article 8). doi: 10.1136/S12913-017-2031-8

Senteio, C and Yoon, D (2020) How primary care physicians elicit sensitive health information from patients. *Qualitative Health Research, 30* (9). doi: 10.1177/1049732320911630

Sharp, S, McAllister, M and Broadbent, M (2016) The vital blend of clinical competence and compassion: how patients experience person-centred care. *Contemporary Nurse, 52* (2–3): 300–12.

Skundberg-Kletthagen, H, Wangenstein, S, Hall-Lord, M et al. (2014) Relatives of patients with depression: experiences of everyday life. *Scandinavian Journal of Caring Sciences, 28* (3): 564–71.

Smith, L (2017) *Meet Maslow: How Understanding the Priorities of Those Around Us Can Lead to Harmony and Improvement.* Scotts Valley, CA: Create Space Independent Publishing.

Sustersic, M, Gauchet, A, Foote, A et al. (2017) How best to use and evaluate patient information leaflets given during a consultation: a systematic review of literature reviews. *Health Expectations, 20* (4): 531–42. doi: 10.1111/hex.12487

Swanwick, T and Vaux, E (2020) *ABC of Quality Improvement in Healthcare.* Chichester: Wiley Blackwell.

Talking Sense (2018) *Counselling for Depression: Rotherham, Doncaster and South Humber NHS Foundation Trust.* Improving Access to Psychological Therapies (IAPT). Available online at: www.talkingsense.org/how-we-can…therapy/…therapy/counselling-for-depression

Teeri, S, Leino-Kilpi, H and Valimaki, M (2016) Long-term nursing care of elderly people: identifying ethically problematic experiences among patients, relatives and nurses in Finland. *Nursing Ethics.* doi: 10.1191/0969733006ne830oa

Thevarajan, I, Buising, K and Cowie, B (2020) Clinical presentation and management of Covid-19. *Medical Journal of Australia.* doi: 10.5694/mja2.50698

Toluwalese, A, Shaw, D and Edwards, K (2019) Feasibility and effectiveness of a mnemonic approach to teach residents how to assess goals of care. *Journal of Palliative Medicine, 22* (6). doi: 10.1089/jpm.2018.0509

Tripathy, N (2019) *Holistic Nursing: Holism and Holistic Health Care for Nurses.* London: Skinny Bottle Publishing.

Turnbull, A, Sahetya, S, Biddison, E et al. (2018) Competing and conflicting interests in the care of critically ill patients. *Intensive Care Medicine, 44*: 1628–37.

Van Belle, E, Gieson, J, Conroy, T et al. (2019) Exploring person-centred fundamental nursing care in hospital wards: a multisite ethnography. *Journal of Clinical Nursing.* doi: 10.1111/jocn.15024

Van der Aa, H, Van Rens, G, Comijs, H et al. (2015) Stepped care for depression and anxiety in visually impaired older adults: multicenter randomized controlled trial. *British Medical Journal, 351*: h6127. doi: 10.1136/bmj.h6127

Van Veer-Tazelaar, P, Van Marwijk, H, Van Oppen, P et al. (2009) Stepped-care prevention of anxiety and depression in late life: a randomized controlled trial. *Archives of General Psychiatry, 66* (3): 297–304.

Warmington, S (2020) *Storytelling Encounters as Medical Education: Crafting Relational Identity.* London: Routledge.

Webster, R, Thompson, A, Norman, P and Goodacre, S (2017) The acceptability and feasibility of an anxiety reduction intervention for emergency department patients with non-cardiac chest pain. *Psychology Health and Medicine, 22* (1): 1–11.

Weiner, B (2010) The development of an attribution-based theory of motivation: a history of ideas. *Educational Psychologist, 45* (1): 28–36.

Weiner, S and Schwartz, A (2016) *Listening for What Matters: Avoiding Contextual Errors in Health Care.* Oxford: Oxford University Press.

Welch, E (2018) *The NHS at 70: A Living History.* Barnsley: Pen and Sword History.

Wilson, L, Tripkovic, L, Hart, K et al. (2017) Vitamin D deficiency as a public health issue: using vitamin D2 or vitamin D3 in future fortification strategies. *The Proceedings of the Nutritional Society, 76* (3): 392–9.

Yao, Y, Wang, H and Liu, Z (2020) Expression of ACE2 in airways: implications for Covid-19 risk and disease management in patients with chronic inflammatory respiratory diseases. *Clinical and Experimental Allergy*. doi: 10.1111/cea.13746

Yehudia, A (2020) 'You're the best nurse I ever had'. *Nursing, 50* (5): 46–7.

Zhou, F, Yu, T, Du, R et al. (2020) Clinical course and risk factors for mortality of adult inpatients with Covid-19 in Wuhan China: a retrospective cohort study. *The Lancet, 395* (10229): 1054–62.

Ziebland, S, Chapple, A and Evans, J (2015) Barriers to shared decisions in the most serious cancers: a qualitative study of patients with pancreatic cancer treated in the UK. *Health Expectations, 18* (6): 3302–12.

Zirak, M, Ghafourifard, M and Mamaghani, E (2017) Patients' dignity and its relationship with contextual variables: a cross-sectional study. *Journal of Caring Sciences, 6* (1): 49–57.

Index

Locators in **bold** refer to tables and those in *italics* to figures.

Milton Keynes UK
Ingram Content Group UK Ltd.
UKHW030408101123
432288UK00001B/2

9 781529 752915